WITHDRAWN

LONGMAN BUILDING STUDIES

Primary Health Care Centres

THE LIBRARY
GUILDFORD COLLEGE
of Further and Higher Education

LONGMAN BUILDING STUDIES

Primary Health Care Centres

A review of current trends and the future
demands for community-based
health care facilities

Martin S. Valins
BA (HONS) DIP ARCH RIBA

71031

725.5
VAL
Not to be taken away

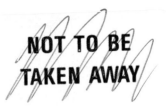
NOT TO BE
TAKEN AWAY

Longman Group UK Limited
Longman House, Burnt Mill, Harlow
Essex CM20 2JE, England
and Associated Companies throughout the world

© Martin S. Valins 1993

Copublished in the United States with
John Wiley & Sons, Inc., 605 Third Avenue,
New York, NY 10158

All rights reserved; no part of this publication may
be reproduced, stored in a retrieval system, or
transmitted in any form or by any means, electronic,
mechanical, photocopying, recording or otherwise,
without either the prior written permission of the
publishers, or a licence permitting restricted copying
in the United Kingdom issued by the Copyright
Licensing Agency, Ltd, 90 Tottenham Court Road,
London W1P 9HE.

First published in 1993

British Library Cataloguing in Publication Data

A CIP record for this title is available from the British Library

Library of Congress Cataloging-in-Publication Data

A CIP record for this title is available from the Library of Congress

ISBN 0 582 09383 X

Produced by Longman Singapore Publishers (Pte) Ltd.
Printed in Singapore

This book was inspired by, and is dedicated to, the
memory of

Dr Ruth Cammock, MD, RIBA (10 Jan 1922–29 July 1989)
Dr Huw C. Davies, MB BCh, MRCGP, DObstRCOG
(6 March 1943–30 Sept 1986)
Dr Donald MacKay, MB CHB, BScHons, FRCGP, DipObs
(25 Sept 1948–14 April 1990)

each of whom contributed to furthering the field of
knowledge in architecture for primary health care.

In architecture as in all other operative arts, the end must direct the operation. The end is to build well. Well building hath three conditions. Commodity, firmness and delight.

Henry Wotton (1568–1639) English poet and diplomat, *Elements of Architecture Part 1*

Health is a precious thing, and the only one, in truth, meriting that a man should lay out, not only his time, sweat, labour and goods, but also his life itself to obtain it.

Montaigne *Of the Resemblance of Children to their Fathers* Essays (1580–88), trans Charles Cotton and W. C. Hazlitt

Contents

Forewords

The moment at which this book appears finds the two professions with which it is concerned in a state of greater uncertainty than at any time since the Second World War.

In the UK at least, after what in retrospect now seem like years of relative stability, the worlds of medicine and architecture have seen their underlying claims of expertise and neutrality thrown into question, their share and long-standing service ethic superseded by the 'enterprise culture'.

The rise in the 'market model' is changing not only the language of the professions but the whole institutional infrastructure through which their activities are conducted. An ideology that regards good health as a 'commodity' to be purchased by 'consumers' is the same ideology that perceives architecture not as an agent of social betterment but as an asset of real estate.

At the same time – and more promisingly – the sceptical scrutiny by 'outsiders' of some form of the more deeply ingrained professional assumptions is forcing medical and architectural practitioners to dismantle many of the self-imposed barriers between themselves and those they purport to serve.

Quite how these emergent trends will develop is far from clear, but it may be predicted that any worthwhile advance can only arise from a deeper understanding of the circumstances from which they grow.

For these very reasons there can surely be no better juncture for the kind of systematic analysis of recent and current practice that is undertaken by this book. Here, in place of the sterile political polarization of so much medical debate or the stylistic name-tagging of most architectural commentary, is a real investigation of contemporary achievement – ranging from informed international comparison to detailed evaluation of individual projects.

If there is one predominant message that emerges from this wealth of material it is that the quality of results is intimately dependent on the quality of dialogue between those involved in their realization, and that this dialogue itself must be informed by an awareness of what is happening on the wider front. The buildings themselves become the living record of this crucial formative process of discussion, interrogation, reflection and, hopefully, progressive mutual enlightenment.

Yet as many established authorities, consultancies and departmental teams are being wound up and dispersed it is precisely this sort of continuous discourse that is interrupted. It is therefore books such as this one that must become the repositories of the cumulative experience and lessons learnt 'in the field', providing both information and inspiration for those seeking to develop the state of the art of architecture for primary health care.

Like any sourcebook it must be questioned, pondered, applied and no doubt in due course updated. In this service it should prove a real benefit not only to the myriad professionals involved, but, as a result, to that even larger interest group that ultimately includes all others – the patients.

John Allan, Director,
Avanti Architects

This book is about change – a necessary and natural change from institutionalized hospital-based health care to a more decentralized, accessible, personalized health care. The change is both required and welcome; acute financial pressures require hospitals to consolidate expensive specialized service while decentralizing primary care; human beings welcome more humane health care environments. Primary health care strips away the bureaucracy and anonymity of the institutional hospital. It is accessible and personalized, the first contact a patient has with the health system.

Benefits to the patient are many: medical costs are reduced; medical services are close to home; doctor/patient confidentiality and trust are strengthened; and overall wellness/preventive medicine practices are more accessible. Similarly, staff prefer primary care facilities because of less hierarchy and greater personal accountability.

Martin Valins provides an international overview of primary health care. Case studies from six countries show both private and socialized medicine in a period of transition towards a more consumer-based health care. While dimensional statistics and regulatory requirements for design and construction vary by region, basic organizational components share the priority that primary health care centres are flexible places for people, not encasements for equipment.

Primary Health Care Centres is an excellent reference for the professional library. It gives an overview of the origins and need for primary care centres and the evolving role of the hospital to provide only highly specialized, highly equipment-intensive medical and in-patient care. The book offers a consolidation of ideas and concise guidelines about critical design issues in primary care facilities.

Thomas P. Spies
Senior Vice President
Cochran, Stephenson & Donkervoet Architects Inc.

Acknowledgements

I am particularly indebted to the following firms of architects whose buildings and projects form the core of this book. I thank them for giving up many hours of their time and offering highly practical and relevant information based upon many years of experience in the field:

Arkkitehtitomisto
Laiho-Pulkkinen-Raunio
Turka, Finland

Associated Architects
Birmingham, England

Avanti Architects Ltd
London, England

Broome Oringdulph
O'Toole Rudolf Boles
& Associates PC (BOOR/A)
Portland, Oregon, USA

Cassidy Taggart
Partnership
Chartered Architects,
Planners & Designers
London, England

Douglas Stephen &
Partners
Chartered Architects
London, England

Drover Welch & Lindlan
DWL Architects &
Planners Inc
Phoenix, Arizona, USA

Joe J. Jordan/Wallace
Roberts & Todd
Architecture, Landscape
Architecture, Urban
Design, Environmental
Planning
Philadelphia, USA

Kirkham Michael &
Associates
Architects – Engineers –
Planners
Omaha, Nebraska, USA

Media Five Ltd
Architecture – Graphic
Design – Interior Design –
Planning – Programming
Honolulu, Hawaii, USA

Parker & Scott Architects
Belfast, Northern Ireland

Karsten Vibild MAA
Køge, Denmark

Penoyre & Prasad
London, England

Robert D. Lynn Associates
Architects, Engineers,
Planners
Philadelphia, USA

Rock Townsend
London, England

Tony Atkin & Associates
Philadelphia, USA

White Arkitekter AB
Stockholm, Sweden

Yasumitsu Matsunaga/
SKM
Architects & Planners
Tokyo, Japan

I would like to acknowledge the contributions of Joe Jordan, FAIA (Wallace Roberts & Todd, Philadelphia, USA), John Allan (Avanti Architects, London, UK), Stephen Gage (Douglas Stephen & Partners, London, UK), Dr Christopher Hindley (Highgate Group Practice, London, UK), Professor

Raymond Moss (MPA, London, UK), and Derek Salter (Care Design Group) who were kind enough to share their experiences in Chapter 5.

Many thanks to the following for their invaluable help:

United States of America
Jenny Hamilton (TAA), Philadelphia, Pennsylvania
Julie Baker (BOOR/A), Portland, Oregon
Gary Dubas, HDR Inc., Omaha, Nebraska
Ron Starr/Lightwaves, San Francisco, California
Greg Scott, Reese Lower Patrick & Scott – Architects, Lancaster, Pennsylvania
Glen Tipton, Cochran Stevenson & Donkervoet, Architects/Interior Designers, Baltimore, Maryland
Richard W. Stephan, New Season Corporation, Jenkintown, Pennsylvania
Ginger Tippie, Director, Office of Educational Services, American Association of Homes for the Aging, Washington DC
Ken Bast, Hamilton/KSA, Minneapolis, Minnesota

Japan
Hiroshi Ijiji, Secretary General Japan Institute of Architects

England and Wales
King's Fund Centre Library & staff, London
Tony Noakes, Architect, Department of Health, London
Lane Whittlesey (Business Consultants), Woking, Surrey
Paul Collinge, Aldington Craig & Collinge, Architects, Bucks
Maritz Vandenberg, London
Michael Francis, Michael Francis Associates, London
Care Design Group, London
The RIBA Library & staff
The Hulton Picture Library, London
Ann Coppinger, Bloomsbury Health Authority
Malcolm Potter, Chief Architect, London Borough of Camden
Ms Edith Fawcett, Sheffield
Mrs Elizabeth MacKay, Cambs
Mrs Rosemary Rubin, Cardiff

Scotland
David Sutherland, Camphill Architects, Aberdeen

Finland
Helina Kotilainen, Laakintohallitus, National Board of Health, Helsinki

Denmark
Mogens Fischer, Det Kongelige Danske Kunstakademi

Sweden
Hakan Olsson, Hakan Estates
Desmond O'Gorman, SPRI, Swedish Planning & Rationalization Institute for Health & Social Services, Stockholm

Germany
R. J. Sahl, BDA Dusseldorf BDA, Munich

Special thanks to my dear parents, Maisie and Hymie Valins, for their support and wisdom. Elaine and Craig Span for help during my stay in the United States. Raymond Valins and Martin Lukover for the valued friendship. Linda Valins for her help in research and administration.

September 1978
Alma-Ata, USSR

A distinguished assembly of health care
professionals and government representatives
assembled to declare their intentions to improve
the health of their peoples so that by the year 2000
reasonable health conditions would prevail
throughout the world. They also agreed a policy to
encourage a move away from concerns purely
medical towards a broader concept of health care
delivery.

This assembly was the 1978 International
Conference of the World Health Organization and
UNICEF which focused on primary health care. It
was one of the first such major international
conferences specifically to discuss primary health
care. The 'Alma-Ata Declaration' as it became
known, placed primary health care high on the
agenda of future change and direction for health
care services throughout the world.

This book is about some of the new building
types that are evolving to accommodate primary
health care services. Whilst examples are drawn
from the United Kingdom, United States, Japan,
Sweden, Denmark and Finland, the information
applies to a far wider international context.

Definitions

A primary health care centre provides a range of
health care services including:

- Medical consultations
- Treatment/diagnostics
- Minor surgery
- Health education

In some instances services may also include:

- Day care for physiotherapy and occupational
  therapy
- Out-patients' emergency treatment

And in some examples:

- In-patient short-stay beds

Primary health care may be described as a nation's
'first line of defence' in maintaining the health and
well-being of its people. Its services would often be
the first (primary) contact a patient has with a
country's health services system. Additional
facilities may be provided for hospital consultants to
hold out-patient sessions within the centre. Other
organizations, such as local self-help groups,
family therapy and child guidance, may also
occasionally use such a centre. It can therefore be
defined as all those services provided outside a
hospital by family doctors, dentists, retail
pharmacists, opticians and other health care
professionals allied to health care working in a
community setting.

Most primary health care centres would have a
core of staff working from the centre which would
include:

- General medical practitioners/physicians
- Health visitors
- Nurse practitioners
- Community and district nurses
- Community physicians
- Administrative staff and managers

In addition there may be other either permanent or
visiting staff using the centre such as:

- Midwives
- Chiropodists
- Therapists
- Dentists
- Specialist consultants
- Physiotherapists
- Occupational therapists
- Opticians
- X-ray lab technicians

The above list is not exhaustive.

The concept of this building type is to encourage,
both through management and design, the active
co-operation of the various medical and social
disciplines, the result of which is to provide a
community-based health care resource providing a
co-ordinated and holistic health care service.

Because this is still both a comparatively new and

evolving building type terminology differs between funding authorities and countries, although the concept remains similar. For example, such buildings have been called:

- Health Centre
- Group Practice Surgery
- Medical Centre
- Ambulatory Care Centre

- Physicians' Clinic
- Medical Office building
- Doctors' Offices

A primary care centre would tend to serve an average local population of between 10,000 and 35,000 people. Generally the centres would operate as a day care facility, although there are models evolving incorporating overnight-stay beds.

The two great professions of medicine and architecture each have their own proud histories of achievement, scientific and technical advances and the overwhelming desire to improve the well-being of the human experience.

The interface between the two occurring in the buildings designed to accommodate and facilitate the practice of medicine can therefore generate a dynamic fusion in the pursuance of professional excellence. History has taught us, however, that it can also often lead to a clash of two established cultures.

During the latter part of the 19th and for the majority of the 20th century it has been the hospital which has become firmly established as the main focus of medical skills and has therefore been the focal point of dialogue between architecture and medicine. Because of their specialist skills, staff resources and technical facilities, hospitals remain vitally important to the delivery of a nation's health care service.

Nevertheless, in post-industrial societies growing attention is now being paid to the concept of providing health care in the community. Architecture for primary health care is therefore an increasingly important and evolving aspect of both medicine and architecture.

Health care in the community

An analysis of many of the health care systems throughout the world bears witness to a change in emphasis away from the provision of large hospitals towards smaller, satellite facilities situated within local communities. This is in response to the almost universal economic crisis in funding large hospital programmes, and has coincided with advances in technologies of health care and preventive medicine.

However, the economic arguments for reducing capital and revenue expenditure on hospitals can only be sustained if there is first the establishment of an adequate infrastructure of such community-based primary care facilities.

These economic and technological factors have also reinforced the recognition that there are social and medical benefits for patients in taking services such as non-acute and out-patient care out of hospitals and into the community. For example, in the United Kingdom the concept of health care in the community has been embraced by successive governments, largely perhaps for its apparent economic savings of public expenditure on centralized resources.

As a reflection of these changes, opportunities have been created for new forms of architecture for primary health care. It has also created the opportunity for a new format of dialogue between contemporary medicine and architecture within a community-based context.

A primary care facility as part of the community fabric

Smaller yet community-based facilities allow for a greater integration and identification within the local community. They can offer an improved access and availability of medical care incorporating the needs and requirements of the patient as a local user/resident. Many of the activities within the centre will largely depend upon patients accepting invitations to attend, for example, preventive medicine programmes. Such programmes will therefore stand a better chance of success in an environment designed to be accessible, welcoming and comfortable.

Contrast with the institution of the hospital

Primary care centres therefore offer both medical and architectural practitioners the chance to break away from the often negative images of the hospital which at worst was typified by the 19th-century hospital building and arguably not much improved during the construction programmes of the 1960s. Because of its sheer size and scale it became almost the cathedral of medicine; patients and junior staff would pass in awe through the anonymous corridors where unfamiliar sounds and smells reinforced a sense of alienation from the medical staff. Despite (or even because of) often chronic under-funding in the public sector, many such hospitals remain (with some lost dignity) inappropriate environments for the delivery of good medicine. In certain instances when located in a hospital campus, the primary care centre can form a bridge between the community and the services of the hospital on a more human scale.

Primary care: a wider definition

Whilst our increasing knowledge and understanding of health care has eradicated certain forms of disease, new forms of health dysfunction have come into focus. Conditions such as AIDS and anorexia nervosa/bulimia, largely unheard of before, now present the challenge of new forms of treatment and care.

The nature of such conditions also require new forms of appropriate health care environments, preferably placed within a community rather than a hospital setting. In recognition of this, two of the buildings and projects to be discussed are deliberately drawn from the outer fringes of the definition of primary care: The Renfrew Center, Philadelphia, for the treatment of anorexia and bulimia (page 68) and the Masku Centre in Finland, caring for patients with multiple sclerosis (page 139).

The book is intended to present an overview of recent significant projects so as to discuss current trends and future directions. It is concerned with the principles of good design and so should be applicable across a whole range of primary care centres. That is, from the smaller single doctor's surgery to large and complex multi-facility centres.

Each building and project study has been selected to illustrate different approaches and design solutions to the provision of primary care facilities. These case studies offer a wide range of options which are analysed within a context of design and functional content and the project's relevance to wider applications and future trends. There are of course numerous examples worthy of inclusion and recognition. Any omission is therefore a reflection of the procedures of selection and certainly not a rejection of quality and achievement. As with any building, each scheme will have its own virtues and deficiencies. They should be viewed with the recommendations of the text in mind.

The book is for those who fund, manage, use and design primary health care facilities. It is therefore addressed to architects and the requirements of health services managers, medical, social and nursing staff and, most importantly, the patients who use the facilities.

Primary Health Care Centres has been laid out first to introduce the broad subject area within an historical context, then to set out the design criteria from which to appraise and analyse the 18 building and project studies. Finally the book concludes with a discussion on possible future directions.

A historical context can bring a rationale to the present situation and produce a basis from which to appraise current trends and future directions.

This chapter describes how the concept for a new building type which was to house the activities of primary health care evolved. The evolution of what was termed 'the health centre' in the United Kingdom was to lay the foundation internationally for the modern primary health care centre.

R. Sand in his 1952 publication *Advance to Social Medicine*[1] traces how the idea of the primary health care centre developed throughout the world from 1900 onwards. It sprang from the basic realization that the various agencies and professions concerned with primary health care could work better if contained within one building. This also included the guiding principle that curative and preventive aspects of medical care are inseparable.

In the United Kingdom, along with most European countries, a glimpse into the history of primary care buildings reveals that an important ancestor of the modern health centre is in fact not a building at all but a market stall. For it was here that the apothecaries practised and traded their medical wares in the market-place of medieval Britain. Because of the non-acute nature of primary care it was usually delivered by a diverse assortment of personnel including no lesser than witches, faith healers and the occasional kindly monk. Yet here are the beginnings of the primary health care team. In an apothecary we see the forerunner of the family doctor, in the kindly monk the health visitor; in the witches, paradoxically, the role of the midwife; and in the faith healer perhaps the role of the community social worker, although it has to be stated that the image of midwives as witches was not unconnected with a conspiracy by the male-dominated medical professions.

In the United Kingdom medicine became more scientific and more established as a profession during the 16th century. As a consequence royal colleges were formed: the Surgeons' in 1540, the Physicians' in 1551 and in 1617 the apothecaries organized and founded their royal college. With

royal patronage these societies were able to wield great political power and influence the further development of medical services and facilities.

For the apothecary the market stall was abandoned for the security and status of the Georgian residence. Indeed during Britain's Golden Age during the mid to late 19th century, the family doctor became a highly respected member of middle class society. His practice was his home simply because all that was required in order to conduct his business was a room, and the nature of the work and the demands of his patients required him to be available throughout the day and night, that is for those who could afford his services, for although a primary health care services was evolving for the middle class, the poor still relied upon charity and hope.

Indeed by the turn of the century health care was still financed and organized by local charities, benefactors and rich industrialists, so that the dispersion of hospitals and any form of health care was located near large population clusters and related very much to the economic status of the local population and not necessarily to need.

As Abel Smith said, 'The pattern of provision depended on the donations of the living and the legacies of the dead rather than any ascertained need.[2]

With the development of labour movements born out of the industrial revolution, workers clubs and friendly societies organized insurance schemes to provide some medical cover. These schemes led to an increase in demand for improvements in the quality of health care and for an extension of insurance cover to include larger sections of the population.

However it was not until 1911 that central government began to respond to this need with the introduction of a National Insurance Bill.

This was in effect until 1948, and under this Bill the central health committee and local insurance committees were established. Additional medical offers of health were appointed and health visitors employed in the field of health education, an area of work the medical profession had ignored in the

CHAPTER **2**

Architecture for primary health care: looking back

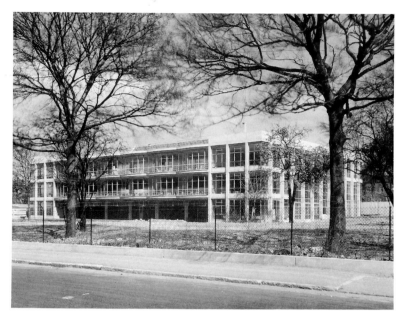

past. A registration of births became obligatory in 1915 and provided health visitors with information so that health education could be carried out in the home.

The social effects of World War I provided a change of values in the medical profession and society generally, which looked for improvements in education, housing and life-style. The local government board circular of 1918 offered grants of up to 50% towards preventive services including the expenses of a 'health centre' which was defined at the time as 'An institution providing any or all of the following activities: medical supervision and advice for expectant mothers and of children under five years of age, and medical treatment at the centre for cases needing it'.[3]

The preventive ideology is emphasized, but the doctor is not mentioned. This was the beginning of the separate local health authority function. At this

△ *The Peckham Health Centre, 1936. Designed by: Sir Owen Williams. Recognized as an innovative model health centre both in its design, structure as well as its medical philosophy.*

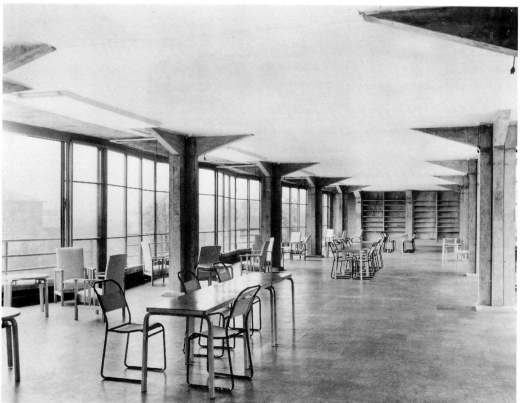

▷ *Interior of dining area, Peckham Health Centre.*

time the general practitioner did not equate with the concept of preventive medicine. From this background the Ministry of Health set up a consultative council on medical and allied services with Lord Dawson of Penn as its chairman in 1920, and it is in this report that the health centre concept is first mentioned as a building type. The Dawson Report as it became known gave details of the type of accommodation (which included ward blocks and X-ray facilities) that would be provided.[4]

When the Dawson committee produced its findings in 1920 they were far in advance of their time. In effect they were advocating a merger of various medical services, preventive and curative, which were on the whole in a very rudimentary stage of development. There was at the time very little co-operation or co-ordination between the different branches of medicine and health care and there was little goodwill. General practice was divided into 'panel' and 'private' with considerable differences in the services which were often competitive. Hospitals did the best they could despite often being starved of money. Local authorities emerged with the best record in that they set up infant welfare, maternity and school health services free to the public, which did not carry total favour with the general practitioners.

In these circumstances it is not surprising that the Dawson Report, made at the urgent request of the government of the day, failed to make any real impact on the profession, and no action was subsequently taken. However, the basic ideas continued to stimulate serious study within the profession from 1930 onwards. While little was done to implement the Dawson Report, the 1930s witnessed two notable exceptions which must stand as one of the first examples of architecture for a more community-based health care facility.[5] The Peckham Health Centre was first opened in 1935. The main aims of its founders Scott Williamson and Innes Pearse were to study the health of a geographically-defined population and to improve the people's health and social functioning. Peckham embodied a holistic view of health which encompassed diet, social and psychological factors.

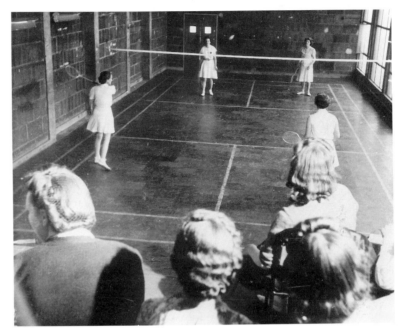

△ *Peckham Health Centre. The centre is used as a social community centre with extensive programmes including dancing, shows and sports programmes.*

▽ *Self-service cafe at Peckham Health Centre. While the centre embodied the philosophy of health and fitness, it is interesting to note that this was prior to a greater consciousness with* *regard to high cholesterol foods and the dangers of smoking. (Picture courtesy of the Hulton-Deutsch Collection.)*

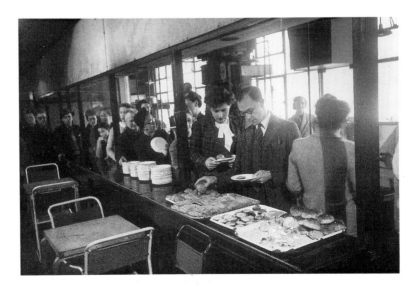

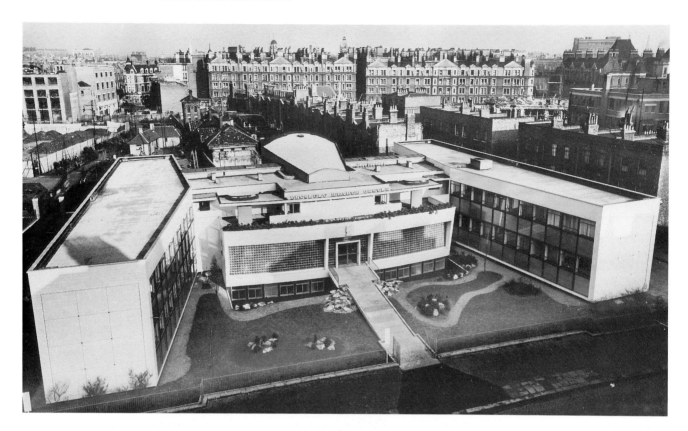

△ The Finsbury Health
Centre, London, 1938.
Architect: Berthold
Lubetkin and the Tecton
group. This provided a
variety of primary health
care facilities from general
practitioner surgeries to
recreational therapy rooms
under one roof.

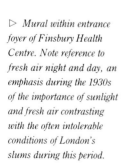

▷ Mural within entrance
foyer of Finsbury Health
Centre. Note reference to
fresh air night and day, an
emphasis during the 1930s
of the importance of sunlight
and fresh air contrasting
with the often intolerable
conditions of London's
slums during this period.

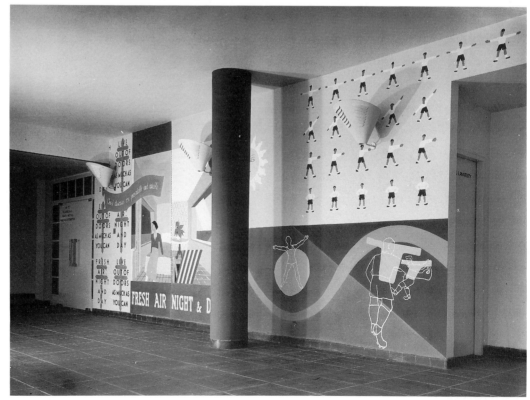

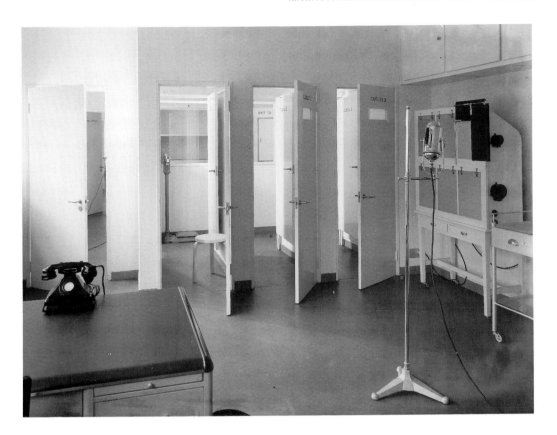

◁ *Interior of clinical area, Finsbury Health Centre.*

◁ *Typical signage of Finsbury Health Centre interior with the promotion of health services.*

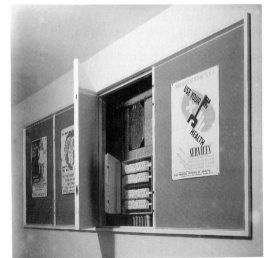

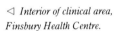

The Peckham Health Centre was perhaps the most expansive in its philosophy and definition of health care. The Centre was used as a social community centre with extensive programmes including dancing, shows, etc. Its ambitious social and medical programme, however, failed to attract adequate financial support. Its doors were eventually closed in 1950.

The second example has however survived from the same experimental period. The Finsbury Health Centre, completed in 1938 and designed by Berthold Lubetkin and the Tecton group, provided a variety of primary health care facilities from general practitioner surgeries to recreational therapy rooms under one roof. Funding is currently being established by the health authority for the building's restoration by Avanti Architects to return it to its former glories.

The Finsbury Health Centre stands as a rare example of the combination of the philosophies of contemporary medicine and architecture, to provide an almost faultless harmony of expression in function and design. As John Allan of Avanti Architects has stated:

As a manifesto of social ideals it affirms an essential proposition which humane architecture can never ignore.[6]

Just as the Peckham and Finsbury Health Centres can be viewed as milestones in the development of architecture of community and primary health care, the Medical Planning Commission of 1942 was seen as a further endorsement of the Dawson Report and became an internationally acknowledged document advocating the concept of the health centre. This body recognized that there was too much diffusion of responsibility for health among various statutory authorities and very little organization within general practice and recommended that:

Each family or individual should be in care of a medical practitioner who shall be concerned not only with diagnosis and treatment but also with prevention of disease. It involves integration of the preventative and personal health services, it also involves radical changes in the country's administrative machinery and in the training of medical students. It assumes that fusion of public health and other forms of practice will result in practitioners in every field working in close contact and accord not only with each other but also with dentists, nurses, midwives, sanitary inspectors and other auxiliaries.[7]

The Commission suggested that for general practitioner services, health centres as defined by the Dawson Committee would be the means of achieving these ends and went on to describe in detail how these should be organized.

Following the National Health Service Act of 1946, the establishment of a National Health Service in the United Kingdom became an admired model throughout the world. It relied upon a compulsory national insurance scheme paid by all tax payers according to income from which the entire nation benefited from free delivery of all health services. The health centre was to become the focal point in the concept of a National Health Service for it was here that it was hoped to make a balance between the functions of a hospital and the local authority. Section 21 of the National Health Service Act reads as follows:

It shall be the duty of every local authority to provide, equip and maintain to the satisfaction of the health minister premises which shall be called 'Health Centres'.[8]

Using the United Kingdom as an example it can therefore be argued that the concept of the primary care health centre was born by the recognition and desire of the medical and allied professions to promote and develop more socially and integrated forms of health services. This coincided with a fertile political and financial framework to justify the economic efficiencies of primary health care within the nation's health service.

References

1. Sand, R. (1952) *Advance to Social Medicine*. Staples Press, London.

2. Smith, A. (1964) *The Hospital 1800–1948*. Thames & Hudson, London, p. 405.

3. Local Government Board Circular, 1918.

4. Dawson Report on the Future Provision of Medical Allied Services, 1920. (Reprinted 1950 by King Edward's Hospital Fund for London.)

5. Noakes, T. (1991) Pioneering ways to health. *The Friend*, **149**(2), 41–42.

6. Allan, A. (1988) Finsbury '50' – caring and causality. *The Architectural Review*, June, 50.

7. The Medical Planning Commission, British Medical Association, London, 1942.

8. Section 21, The National Health Service Act, 1946.

Unless otherwise stated photographs in this chapter have been reproduced with the kind permission of the Architectural Press, London.

An analysis of any completed building can only be undertaken with due regard to a whole range of factors, from conceptual to detail, which have played a part in determining the built solution.

Conceptual factors of the political/economic framework of a nation translate into a building's inherent social philosophy. Local regulations, however, also influence and to some extent control design.

Indeed it could be argued that it is sometimes because of the increasing plethora of detail regulations that the conceptual objective of buildings can sometimes become irretrievably compromised.

In formulating a design criteria it is therefore important to establish those basic yet crucial factors which can apply across the international spectrum of primary health care design.

This section of the book provides an activity-led base criteria directly applicable to the design of primary health care centres. It does not lay down specific room sizes or space standards. Invariably these are tied to existing funding methods and national codes and procedures. Instead it is the activities that are described so as to understand why certain criteria are important and not simply how large a room should be.

Correct analysis of building and project studies can then follow as to how an architectural solution has translated function into a coherent form.

Back to basics

The basic design criteria of any primary health care centre will be its ability to facilitate the patient care session, that is, the coming together of a patient (or groups of patients) and a health practitioner within an environment that is accessible and allows for privacy, confidentiality and dignity. This chapter sets out the fundamental principles of primary health care design and then discusses these in relation to organization and management principles upon which the design and function of the building depends for the delivery of effective primary health

care programmes.

Such principles apply to both publicly and privately funded projects since their success is measured by equating the financial resources utilized to develop the project with:

- The efficient delivery of a primary health care service.
- The effective utilization of the building and its services by the patient population being served.
- The facility's ability to attract and retain the best quality medical and administrative staff.

Whatever the social requirements and needs for a particular location are, the public sector demands efficient utilization of often limited financial resources to justify investment. Similarly the private sector will need to seek a return on capital investment in order to provide a viable project.

The design criteria set out below is a response to the needs of the patient and sensitive to the economic equation of financial viability. At best they are in any event inseparable.

Location

A critical factor in the development of any primary health care service will be the quality of the site and its relationship with other community-based facilities. Site selection will bring into play the feasibility of a project from a financial, geographical, technical, planning and design viewpoint. The importance of the site being easily accessible is a simple yet key site location factor.

Primary care – community or hospital-based
Some projects have been developed within the grounds of hospitals. From the medical viewpoint this has advantages in that centralized and expensive technical facilities of a hospital are made easily available for any specialist day-care treatment. The disadvantage is that the building could be perceived as part of the hospital rather than as a community resource. The key factor will be accessibility. Primary care centres (as described in the building and project studies) have become

▷ *Primary health care facility as part of a 'medical park' or 'mall'. From a medical viewpoint the advantage is that the centralized and expensive technical facilities of the hospital are easily available for any specialist day care treatment.*

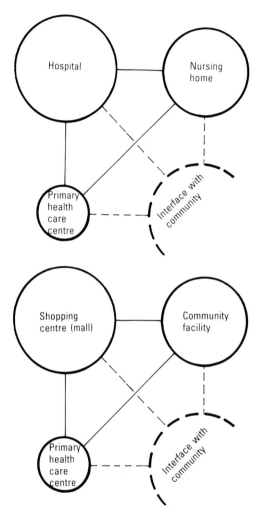

▷ *Primary care facility as part of a community resource, such as a shopping centre or other community buildings. The key factor is accessibility.*

merged with hospital services forming part of a medical 'park' or 'mall', or in other situations the primary care centre becomes integrated with a more community-based facility such as a shopping centre.

Access for physically frail and disabled users
However well a centre is located, its accessibility will still be restricted if due care and attention is not paid to those who may be disabled or physically frail. In the United Kingdom during the past five years, building regulations have rightly imposed mandatory minimum standards for wheelchair user

access to public buildings including primary care centres.

On 26th July 1990 President George Bush signed the Americans with Disabilities Act (ADA) setting out a framework which included compulsory access for the estimated 43 million Americans with physical and mental disabilities for various building types, including medical facilities. The framework of the Act relates not just to visitors of facilities, but also the staff who work in them.

Apart from the internal layout, the route/access to the front door demands particular attention and is not always covered under regulation standards. Demographic profiles of most industrialized nations indicate the increasing numbers of elderly people in relation to the rest of the population. All primary care centres will therefore increasingly be serving an older population. Whilst this will change the demands upon the type of medical services required, it will also focus upon the building to ensure that access for the physically frail is not unnecessarily restricted through insensitive or inappropriate design.

The experience of the patient/visitor
A typical activity sequence for the patient would be:

• Arrival at centre's location
• Entry to the centre
• Confirmation of arrival – reception
• Circulation within the building
• Time spent waiting for patient care session
• Time spent taking part in patient care session
• Departure

Each activity will also involve the successful negotiation of movement around the building from reception to waiting to consultation, and so on.

Entering the centre
A visitor's first experience of the centre, either as a patient or prospective patient, will be the main entrance. The quality of the design and the ease with which a person may negotiate their journey

10

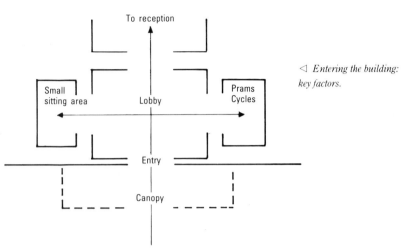

◁ Entering the building: key factors.

into the centre will certainly influence their first impressions.

The main entrance should therefore be clearly visible when first entering the site of the centre to help both first time and regular patients to find their way into the building without confusion. It should be possible to supervise the point of entry to the site visually from the main reception point, both to improve security and make it possible to attend to anyone in difficulty immediately outside the building.

The pedestrian route from the point of entry to the site and to the centre's main entrance should be clearly indicated and segregated from any vehicular traffic route. The route should also be well lit.

While changes in levels are often unavoidable, ramps and gradients should be 1:20 with a maximum of 1:12. However, for those using a walking stick or frame a ramp can often prove difficult and sometimes a hazard. Steps should therefore be provided as well as ramps. Any such facilities should also be accompanied by an easily gripped and visually distinctive handrail.

Design details
- By the use of changes in colour and texture ample warning of any change in level should be clearly indicated.
- The entrance door itself should be clearly perceived and distinguished from any other external doors.
- Door ironmongery should also be easily distinguished and easy to grasp.
- Where possible external doors should not be highly sprung but easy to open.
- At the door set raised thresholds could prove a hazard. Levels on both sides of the front door should therefore be equal.
- A canopy to offer shelter as visitors transfer in and out of vehicles from the main entrance is important. Visitors, especially those less ambulant, may take some time getting in or out of a vehicle.
- Visitors will be reluctant to leave cycles or particularly prams unattended. While an

increasing majority of parents use foldaway devices, an area that can be visually supervised from the waiting area that is secure and sheltered should be provided.
- As there will be a high throughput of patients throughout the day provision of a draught lobby is seen as desirable from the viewpoint of security, heat loss and maintenance of floor finishes.
- Inside the building a small sitting space should be provided with a view out to the main entrance area to enable patients to await the arrival of taxis, etc.
- Also within the lobby area sufficient space should be allocated for notice boards for health education information and community notices. Some visitors may wish, with the management's permission, to pin their own notices, so the boards should be at an easily accessible height.
- A payphone would also be useful for patients wishing to call taxis or, for example, to telephone a friend or relative on the outcome of a consultation/examination.

Confirmation of arrival – reception
Reporting to the reception desk will be the first point of contact for a patient/visitor with a member of staff. In larger facilities the activity of reception may be a two stage process: a general information point and then a secondary reception area located closer to the particular consultation area. The design should allow for the ease of location of the reception area from the main entrance. The reception desk should therefore face directly on to

▷ *Reception desk activities: key factors.*

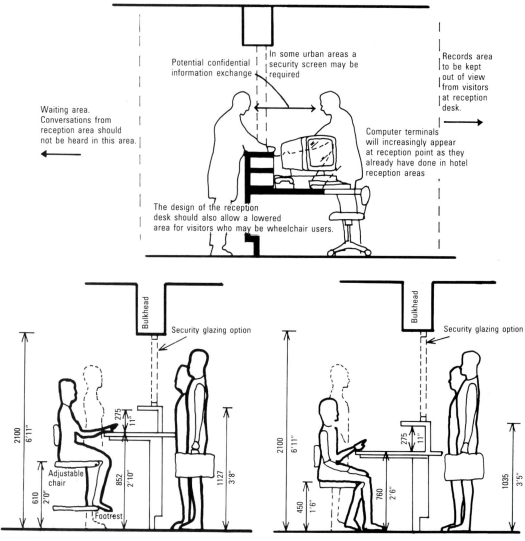

the main entrance area (via the entrance lobby). In this situation visitors are able to see the reception desk from the point of entry, and also the receptionists are able to supervise all those who enter and leave the building.

At each reception point the all important criteria of privacy, confidentiality and dignity will need to be conveyed to the visitor.[1] Confidential information may be shown across the reception desk. The visitor would normally only want to see or hear the receptionist and no-one else during this

exchange of information. Problems of confidentiality may occur if the reception area is, however, located too close to the records and waiting areas. A visitor engaged in conversation with the receptionist should not be able to overlook the records area. In practice this is a common design fault, allowing a multitude of people to overlook and overhear the visitor/patient and receptionist in conversation.

The reception area, because of its public and therefore sometimes vulnerable location, will need to address certain security issues.

Security of information   Patients' records, files and various administrative documents are often located adjacent to the reception desk. They should not, however, be on full display. This might give the impression that records, which all contain confidential information, are not treated as such. In certain areas the security of the reception staff may need to be addressed. In such instances, particularly in inner cities, secure counters as seen in banks may need to be integrated within the design of the desk.

Waiting for consultation/session
From entering the building, reporting to reception and then walking to the waiting room, the activity of waiting marks the most significant period in which the visitor has to assume a passive role and simply sit and wait. Physical passivity, however, belies the ongoing emotional stress and anxiety that continues and even increases when the body is temporarily at rest.

Social psychologist Dr Peter Marsh has compared the experience of waiting to Jean-Paul Sartre's 'Huis Clos', where 'the eternal waiting room in which the characters are stranded represents Hell'.[2]

A waiting space has two main functions

- To provide a convenient point of assembly for patients to consult a member of the health team.
- To provide a restful and non-institutional environment to help reduce a patient's anxiety and so enhance the quality of the impending consultation.

During the time spent in a waiting room the patient/visitor will be able to focus on the centre, its decor, its facilities, etc. This will influence a patient's perception of the efficiency and competence of the centre's administrative and medical staff. However forward thinking, innovative and caring a medical team are, the layout and design of the waiting area will either support or discredit their image. Although each patient will attend the centre for a different reason, it is possible to subdivide waiting patients into the following groups, which may then require different types of waiting spaces.

One-to-one medical consultation   Here the patient may have initiated the consultation by arranging an appointment in response to a problem they wish to discuss with a doctor. The patient may feel extremely anxious about the possible diagnosis, likely treatment and prognosis. The problem could be highly confidential. During the waiting period, therefore, such patients would be unlikely to communicate with other waiting patients. They will be sensitive and may well be easily irritated by other patients coughing, crying babies and worries about cross-infection.

One-to-one treatment consultation   This may well involve a patient who has been invited into the centre, perhaps from a routine screening or as a follow-up treatment after a previous consultation. The patient may therefore be 'well'. The same anxieties may, however, still be present and the need for privacy will still be critical.

Group clinic/session   Here patients will assemble, also perhaps at the invitation of the centre. Each visitor shares a common reason for attending the session (patients attending a Well Baby clinic, for example). Other clinics/session would include a Stop Smoking group or diet classes, or group therapy sessions. Within the containment of the session waiting patients may gain support and comfort by communicating with each other during the waiting period, especially if they are held at regular intervals. The need for privacy is therefore expressed as a group rather than on an individual basis. Clearly it will be inappropriate for all types of waiting patients to be accommodated in the same space at the same time. There is therefore a requirement for a subdivision of waiting spaces in both physical area and time management.

Common to all waiting areas would be the following criteria

- Visual access to the reception area.
- Unobtrusive yet easy access to toilets.

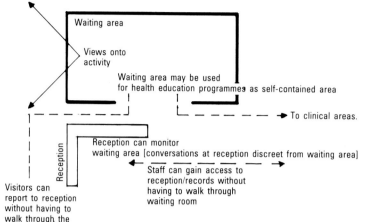

▷ *(a) Waiting area
activity: key relationships.*

- The area should be self-contained with no through circulation to minimize unnecessary disturbance.
- Patients/visitors will spend up to 30 minutes in a waiting space and there is therefore a need to reduce patient boredom and anxiety. Provide ways of distracting them from the activities of the building and from each other: something to look at, such as magazines, the passers-by in the street outside, or the garden. Indeed an American study on architecture and social behaviour[3] has confirmed the importance of such social screens in effectively reducing discomfort and distracting a patient's attention from the presence of others.

Another common feature on the walls of many waiting rooms is the display of various notices – warnings and dangers related to one's health. If one of the functions of a waiting room is to reduce the patient's anxiety before the consultation, this may not be the most appropriate place for such notices, as they can only increase anxiety.

Moving around the building

The function of the circulation spaces in a centre is to provide the most efficient method of connecting space A to space B. More than any other factor, circulation will bring into focus the requirement for clarity and rationality in how a patient moves from one area of the centre to another.

Patients negotiating the circulation areas will often be on their own. They will therefore be relying upon the building design to guide them, without undue stress or confusion, to their destination. Patients may already feel anxious prior to or after their consultation. A major design criteria should therefore be to ensure that the circulation areas do not contribute further to this, and instead allow the patient to move around the building without the anxiety of getting lost or confused.

Circulation distances that are too far will be a nuisance to staff and patients. It may also increase the time between the practitioner calling for the patient from the waiting room and their arrival at the consultation room. This in turn will increase the overall time spent per patient resulting in longer waiting periods.

The slower pace at which many elderly or handicapped patients walk brings into play the importance of paying attention to detailed design of circulation areas.

The image that a centre projects, especially upon one's first visit, will be influenced by the design of the circulation spaces. While financial considerations can lead to a specification which advises a reduction in circulation, even a centre

▽ *(b) Variation in corridor
widths provide node points
to circulation areas.*

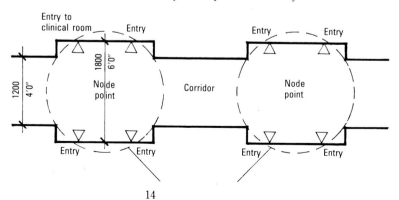

with the most well thought out facilities will appear institutional if the corridors appear utilitarian and passages unrelieved.

Design criteria   The length of any corridor used by a patient should be kept to a minimum, ideally no more than 30 metres (100 ft).

- The width of those corridors used by patients should not be too narrow or uniform in width as this can contribute to an institutional appearance.
- Corridors with variety in their character and width appear to be more successful. Articulation of the corridor space can add meaning to the entrances of the rooms and various spaces.

The introduction of recessed points of entry and clustering of doors achieves a modulation through the corridor which can be reinforced with lighting to accent the point of entry.

This can all contribute significantly to differentiating the corridor spaces.

- A variation in corridor width between 1200 mm (4 ft) and 1800 mm (6 ft) is therefore desirable with the increased width occurring at door entrances creating a focal point, or a clue for orientation.
- The introduction of natural light into corridor spaces although important is not always easy. The most economic solution will favour a double loaded corridor, possibly restricting the opportunity for daylight. One of the successful examples of daylighting a circulation space can be seen at the John Telford Clinic in North East London (further illustrated in the building and projects studies).
- The provision of notice boards and pictures positioned at eye level will add interest to the space while at the same time helping to remind the visitor where they are in relation to the rest of the building.
- The interior finishes of a corridor can help alleviate the institutional qualities associated with corridor design, and can also help distinguish different parts of the building from each other, to break down the scale and avoid uniformity and therefore the possibility of confusion.

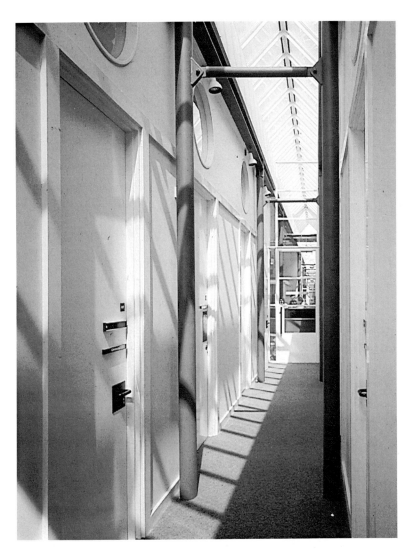

△ *Circulation area at John Telford Clinic. Architects: Avanti Architects Ltd. Photography: Martin Charles.* 'To some extent one's room for manoeuvre is predetermined by the specific attributes of a given site and a given brief. Architecturally we are predisposed to feel that something just called "a corridor" is not a particularly desirable space, yet it has to be said that certain concepts to do with separation and privacy viz-à-viz consulting rooms, waiting areas and so forth can be effectively dealt with by the device of a corridor. Therefore one is looking at a form of space which is joining different functions and looking at what is a positive interpretation of that space. For example, such spaces should, wherever possible, enjoy natural light.' *John Allan, Avanti Architects.*

15

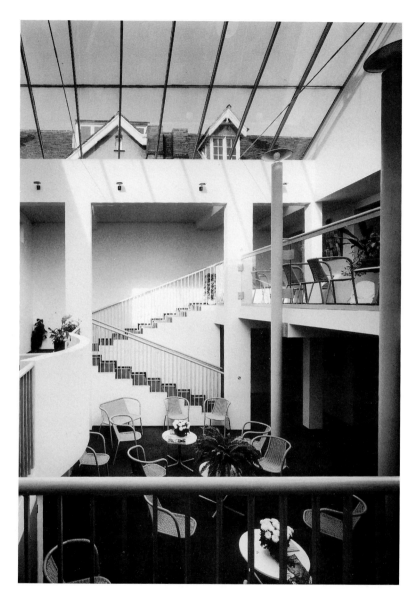

- In schemes with more than one level, floor numbers should be clearly visible from the entry point, i.e. stair or lift lobbies of each floor. As well as the use of colour coding, consideration should also be given to providing landmarks by the lift/stair lobby (i.e. a small sculpture or a painting) to reinforce the identity of each area. As one moves along the corridor the use of paintings or prints as discreet landmarks will help.
- Differentiating wall, ceiling and floors by colour and texture and by picking out features such as skirtingboards and door frames will reduce the possibility of disorientation.
- While the use of fluorescent strip lighting is accepted as the most economical form of lighting, from a maintenance point of view, it can enforce an institutional feel especially when mounted centrally on corridor ceilings. Consideration should be given to other forms of low-energy lighting which may be wall-mounted. Highlighting node points such as entrances also helps to break down the scale of the corridor. However, the lighting design should ensure adequate illumination of all circulation areas once again bearing the elderly patient in mind.
- A key feature of circulation routes will be a handrail fixed on both sides of the corridor at a height of 900 mm (3 ft). For those patients who may have failing eyesight it is important that the handrail is easily distinguishable from the rest of the wall. It should also be easily gripped.

The patient care session

The patient care session will be a major function and purpose of the centre. The main activities involved within such a session include one or more of the following:

- Consultation
- Interview
- Examination
- Treatment and minor surgery
- Group session

In order for each of the above activities to be

△ *Circulation space at Highgate Group Practice. Architects: Douglas Stephen & Partners. Photography: Martin Charles. 'I look towards building forms for primary care where the sterility of the corridor is replaced by a more enlightened approach to how staff and patients move around the building. One should not simply be taking people from spaces and then squeezing them down corridors and into rooms. Concepts involving privacy do not necessarily imply the corridor as an automatic device. Privacy is a concept which is ongoing.' Stephen Gage, Douglas Stephen & Partners.*

effective, the patient needs to be assured that the environment allows for the free flow of confidential information and that this takes place with the utmost privacy and dignity.

Consultation/interview Both these activities are similar in that a patient will be alone with the health practitioner. The patient will be trying to explain the problem, and the health practitioner asking further information and offering advice. It is therefore primarily an activity where the patient and health practitioner engage in a conversation. No surgical procedures normally take place, and the session ends with:

- a diagnosis of the problem and the health practitioner recommending a treatment (i.e. prescribing a medicine).
- the practitioner needing to know more about the problem and requesting that the patient undertakes an examination.
- the health practitioner referring the patient to seek more specialist advice, i.e. a hospital consultant.
- the health practitioner offering a diagnosis to the problem and referring the patient to another member of the health team within the centre (i.e. the nurse) or to a group session.
- the health practitioner offering a diagnosis and requesting that the patient returns for another appointment.

The environment, therefore, does not require any clinical equipment or finishes. Doctors will tend to work from their own consulting rooms and also use this as their administrative base: their office. In the United States doctors would tend to see the patient in an examination room and carry out administrative duties within their own office. Whatever the situation, it should be possible for doctors to impose some of their own tastes within the room. This will help to personalize the space and provide a more informal setting. Indeed, the more patients can be reassured that they are in an informal and safe environment, the greater the chance that they will feel free to express their problem.

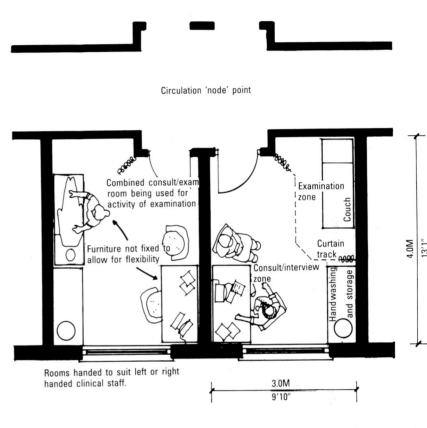

Circulation 'node' point

Combined consult/exam room being used for activity of examination

Furniture not fixed to allow for flexibility

Examination zone

Couch

Curtain track

Consult/interview zone

Handwashing and storage

4.0M 13'1"

Rooms handed to suit left or right handed clinical staff.

3.0M 9'10"

Visual privacy essential: screen wall allows option for daylight to rooms with views onto controlled 'courtyard' area.

Many patients, though presenting a medical symptom, actually seek advice related to a more personal, emotional or sometimes sexual problem. The setting must therefore be conducive to allow the patient to discuss these issues. On occasion the patient may be accompanied by an escort (parent, daughter, spouse, etc.) and with the permission of the patient the doctor may also be accompanied by a medical student to observe the consultation. The room will occasionally therefore need to accommodate these additional numbers, and yet remain an intimate and informal space. Rooms of approximately 12 to 15 sq m (130 to 160 sq ft) appear to satisfy most space requirements.

△ *Diagram of Cedar House Medical Centre combined consulting/ examination room. Architects: Martin Valins & Associates.*

Examination In many respects examination is a continuation of consultation. It will involve the health practitioner either examining a particular symptom or undertaking a more thorough examination to ascertain the general state of health of a patient. Essentially the doctor will be looking/ listening, and as with consultation will need to rely upon the dialogue with the patient to gain as much information as possible. As an investigative procedure there would normally be no requirement for surgical activities and therefore no requirement for clinical finishes. Indeed, as with consultation, the more relaxing the environment, the better chance for an effective examination.

It is desirable that patients have their life functions (blood pressure, pulse etc.) at normal levels prior to examination. Anxiety due to fear generated by a clinical and unfamiliar environment elevates the patient's life functions and may give a false reading.[4]
Jain Malkin

The activities of consultation and examination can therefore be carried out within the room type. Depending upon established methods of working, examinations are sometimes carried out in a separate space.

The advantages of combining consultation and examination within one room are:

- Continuity of contact between doctor and patient, that is, the patient does not have to transfer to a different room to be examined.
- More efficient utilization of building space through the dual function of consultation and examination, thereby saving on both capital and revenue resources for the building project.

There are also disadvantages:

- If a patient takes too long to dress or undress this can unduly increase the session time.
- Some doctors can show a patient to an examination where the nurse may help prepare the patient for the examination while the doctor can attend to another patient (i.e. to improve patient flow). However, design guidance has often under-sized examination rooms, making

them inappropriate for any other use (e.g. a room with a couch only, for use in interviews and consultation).

Cammock, in her pioneering research into the utilization of consulting and examination rooms in United Kingdom health centres, advocated that in the event of separate consulting and examination rooms, these should be designed to a similar space standard.[5] This was to allow for flexibility of use over time, and to respond to the work patterns of medical staff still evolving within an essentially new building type. In essence she argued for more of a loose rather than net fit of room sizes to anticipated functions. (This will be further discussed in Chapter 5.)

Treatment More than any other space within a primary health care centre the function of the treatment room has developed rapidly over the past five years. This is perhaps a reflection of the increasing role of the nurse as a member of the health care team.

The activity of treatment is to carry out procedures as recommended by the doctor and may include the following:

- Injections (vaccination).
- Taking a blood sample.
- Administering a dressing/or redressing.
- Minor surgery (under local anaesthetic in association with other qualified staff).
- Contraceptive (coil, ID) insertions.

In more rural locations where patients may be a greater distance from hospital facilities, the treatment room may also have to offer some accident and emergency treatment. In such cases the treatment suite should have its own entrance to avoid the circulation of emergency patients through the main entrance and circulation areas (see Inscription House, page 60).

In regular treatment sessions the patient will tend already to have been diagnosed, therefore the purpose of the session is the treatment following a consultation/examination by a doctor/physician.

As opposed to the preferably informal setting of the consultation/examination space, the treatment room should reflect the ability to carry out procedures within an efficient and hygienic framework. It should be easy to clean and wash all surfaces. Good overall lighting is essential.

Patients may be required to produce urine samples, therefore a specimen WC (which could double as a disabled patients' WC) should be located adjacent to the treatment room. Using a simple hatch device, the sample can be taken and then passed to the nurse for testing later, either on site or in an off-site laboratory.

Earlier centres saw treatment areas of just one room of approximately 18 sq m (193 sq ft). However, as its importance and function has grown, so the layout of the area has developed into a series of clinical areas with direct access to utility service areas, depending upon the size of the centre.

Within the clinical areas of the treatment room the same requirements for confidentiality, privacy and dignity apply.

Group session   In contrast to the one-to-one session between health practitioner and patient, the facilities of the centre must also allow for groups of people who may share a similar circumstance, including the following:

- Parentcraft.
- Relaxation classes.
- Post-natal classes.
- Eating disorder groups.
- Smokers groups.
- Therapy/counselling group sessions.

While communication within the group may not be as private as in a contained group, patients will require identical criteria for group privacy, confidentiality and dignity. The success of this type of session relies upon the visitor voluntarily attending the session often on a regular basis. The space for group sessions should allow for approximately 12 antenatal patients lying on the floor for relaxation and exercises in preparation for

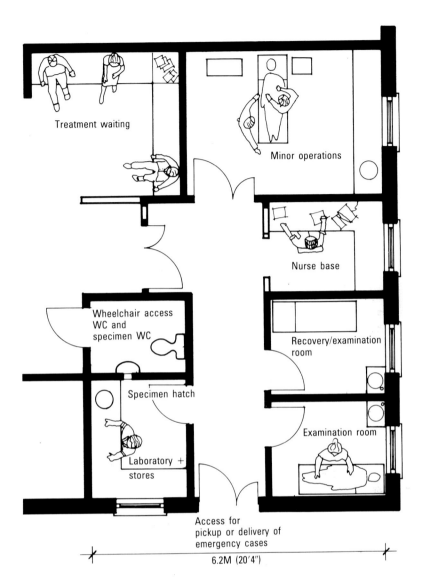

Treatment waiting

Minor operations

Nurse base

Wheelchair access WC and specimen WC

Recovery/examination room

Specimen hatch

Examination room

Laboratory + stores

Access for pickup or delivery of emergency cases

6.2M (20'4")

9.0M
29'6"

birth. This will imply a minimum area of 40 sq m (430 sq ft).

The group space will require:

- Loose furniture to allow for various seating arrangements.
- Access to a small kitchen for the serving of refreshments.
- Access to a store for audio visual equipment, mattresses, etc.
- Complete audio and visual privacy from the rest of the centre's activities.
- As a group space the particular activities of the group may generate noise, so audio privacy will be a two-way constraint.
- If possible the space should be located near the

△ *Layout of treatment room for large general practice medical centre in Dorset, UK. Note the incorporation of a minor operations room plus the facility for alternative access in the case of emergencies which is required because of this centre's remote location from the nearest hospital. Architects: Martin Valins & Associates.*

19

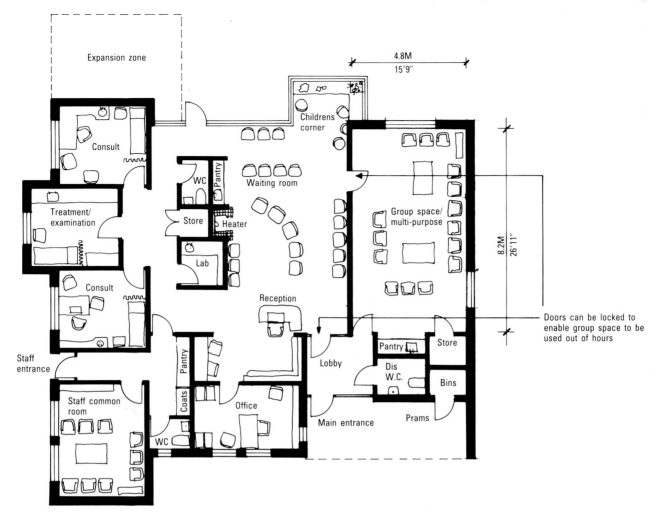

Expansion zone

Consult

Treatment/
examination

Consult

Staff
entrance

Staff common
room

WC

Coats

Pantry

Office

WC

Reception

Lobby

Main entrance

Prams

Bins

Store

Dis
W.C.

Pantry

Group space/
multi-purpose

Doors can be locked to
enable group space to be
used out of hours

8.2M
26'11"

4.8M
15'9"

Childrens
corner

Waiting room

WC

Pantry

Store

Heater

Lab

△ *Layout of smaller
medical centre (238 sq m,
2560 sq ft) illustrating how
in practice the group space
area can function as part
of, or independently from,
the activity of the facility.
Based upon design by J.C.
Clair, Dip.Arch. RIBA.*

main entrance so that arrival and departure of
groups will cause minimal disruption to the rest
of the centre. This will also allow for its use out
of hours if the rest of the building can be secured
beyond the group space. (See Shaw Memorial
Hospital Ambulatory Care Centre, page 34).
It may not be possible to justify an area in the
building exclusively for group sessions. However, a
waiting area may be used for the sessions if it can
satisfy the criteria for privacy. This can be achieved
by designing a waiting area that follows these dual,
yet quite separate activities. Effective time
management of the centre will be needed to
maximize this utilization of space.

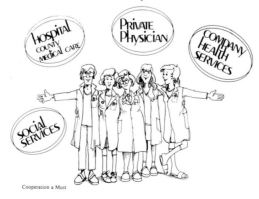

Hospital
County Medical Care

Private
Physician

Company
Health
Services

Social
Services

Cooperation a Must

▷ *Co-operation is a must.
Reprinted with kind
permission of SPRI
(Primary Care in Progress,
p. 11) Stockholm, Sweden,
1984.*

The experience of staff

In order for the patient to benefit from the team
approach to the delivery of a primary health care
service, the building must, through design and
management, encourage opportunities for
collaboration and co-operation between the team
members of staff.

Staff Common Room

An important resource within the centre is a staff
room. This area serves as a place to enjoy a coffee
or meal break. More importantly, it will provide an
area for the various staff members, administrative
and medical, to meet and discuss the workings of
the centre and particular patient programmes.

At times certain staff will meet to review patient
case studies and discuss patient details. Such
activities necessitate adherence to privacy and
confidentiality of conversations and records. As
such, the location of the staff common room
necessitates a complete separation from the patient
areas. Because the activities of a rest area and
those of a space for staff discussing patients may
not be compatible, larger centres tend to have a
staff coffee room adjacent to, but separate from,
the staff lounge. This allows staff to take a coffee

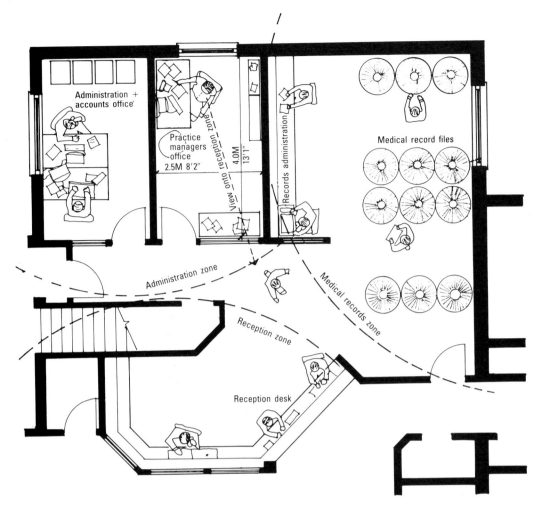

Administration +
accounts office'

Practice
managers
office
2.5M 8'2"

View onto reception zone

4.0M
13'1"

Records administration

Medical record files

Administration zone

Medical records zone

Reception zone

Reception desk

◁ *Layout of administrative
reception and medical
records area at Weavers
Medical Centre, Kettering,
UK. Note how the activities
area of administration,
medical record filing and
reception are zoned to allow
each work function to
remain discreet yet
accessible to the other work
areas.*

break while other staff are engaged in a group
discussion. The sizing of the rooms will depend
upon the anticipated numbers of staff. An
approximate guide, however, is a minimum room of
15 square metres (160 sq ft) with a pro rata
increase of 1.5 square metres (16 sq ft) per member
of staff.

The staff room must also have easy access to:

- Staff WCs.
- Staff changing rooms.
- Pantry/kitchen.

services will demand further administrative areas
for both auditing and the business management.
Senior management will require office space to
interview and hire administrative staff, discuss with
the medical staff potentially confidential
information, etc. Offices will therefore also require
the criteria of privacy and confidentiality while
needing to be quite separate from the patient areas.
Larger centres will require additional administrative
space for secretarial support in the running of the
centre.

Practice manager

The effective management of a centre relies upon
the administrative skills of the practice manager. As
with the role of a nurse, the importance of
management has come sharply into focus,
particularly as the administrative burden and paper
work simply to run a centre have grown
considerably over the past five years.

In the United States administrators' duties have
also involved dealing with patient accounts and the
financial affairs of the centre. In the United
Kingdom, fund holding and new contracts of

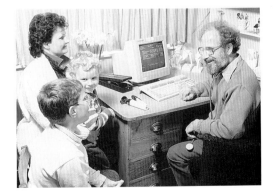

◁ *The implication for
design in relation to the
introduction of new
technology is that computer
terminals will increasingly
appear in the consultation/
examination and treatment
rooms, as well as the
administrative areas.
Photograph supplied
courtesy of AAH Meditel
Ltd. supplier of GP
computer systems.*

Medical records

Efficient storage of medical records will be the major administrative function of the centre. Records must be securely maintained and easy to retrieve. They contain the history of each patient who uses the centre. Through the professional code of conduct doctors are sworn to protect an ethical principle, part of which states that they must not reveal unauthorized information about their patients. The medical records are therefore part of this undertaking. Their use, handling and storage should therefore be treated confidentially.

There are a wide range of methods for storing records. The choice of storage will largely depend upon the records system that the management prefers, but will be influenced by space allocation, etc. Whatever system is adopted, the records will need to be secure from

- unauthorized inspection
- theft
- fire.

In addition, they should be easily accessible to authorized staff in terms of physical reach within a clear system of demarcation. As well as patient medical records, other categories such as age/sex and 'at risk' registers increasingly augment the main records section.

Support areas

In addition to the main areas for staff use, adequate provision is required for the storage of equipment and materials plus support areas for staff changing rooms and wash rooms. A common complaint is the lack of adequate and appropriate storage. The main items for storage are:

- clinical supplies (dressing, incontinence pads, bulk items)
- nursing equipment
- stationery
- furniture not in use.

All storage (particularly clinical supplies and equipment) need to be secure and easily accessed by all members of staff. Adequate provision should also be made for the acceptance of regular deliveries of bulk items.

Information technology

As part of the force to help tackle the increasing amount of information storage within primary care, computer technology has been playing an increasingly vital role.

As with computer technology in general, the major problem has been its sheer pace of development. Today's technological miracle can so often become tomorrow's redundant equipment. There have been two phases in the development of information technology in primary care. The first mainly tackled the administrative chores. Later systems managed clinical information, based upon data from within the centre (patients' clinical details, treatment, etc.). The third phase – the computer and its information – will break out of the building itself and communicate directly with central reference systems, hospitals and, of course, other primary health care centres.

The advent of such technology will give the health care team access to a wider range of information. As such, the terminal will become the major interface of information between the centre and data resources elsewhere. It will play an increasing role in consultation, as an active giver of information rather than as a passive receiver and store of existing data.

For example, if the computer holds information stating that a patient's records include a history of high blood pressure, the system will not return to the menu until the doctor has confirmed that a blood pressure test has been undertaken and that this has been entered into the patient's records. Technology should also allow for greater cross-reference of information between members of the primary health care team, and so increase the opportunities for co-operation in a patient's treatment.

The implication for design is to assume that terminals will increasingly appear in the consultation/examination and treatment rooms as well as the administrative areas. Ducting for cables and designated sources of supply will therefore contribute to the increased service demands of the building.

It can be assumed that as well as the quality of the design and the management of the staff, the ability to utilize information technology will be a major factor in determining the potential of a primary care centre to provide a fully integrated service to its patients.

Relationship of spaces

The primary health care centre relies on an efficient flow of patients and staff through the various spaces in the building. The relationship of those spaces is therefore a critical factor in determining how well a centre can function and maintain the criteria of privacy, confidentiality and dignity.

Following on from the work of Dr Ruth Cammock in her analysis of the spatial relationship of primary health care buildings, it is possible to identify and distinguish three types of territories in any primary care centre within which are the following:

Territory	Typical room/area within each territory
Staff	Records area, common room, administrative office, staff WCs
Public	Patient entrance/waiting area
Patient care	Consultation, interview, examination, group space, and any other room used for patient care sessions

As Cammock explains in her book *Primary Health Care Buildings*

The more clearly the building can reflect this distinction the better it will meet the needs of both groups.[6]

The arrangement of spaces should allow staff and patients to circulate without unscheduled or inappropriate contact.

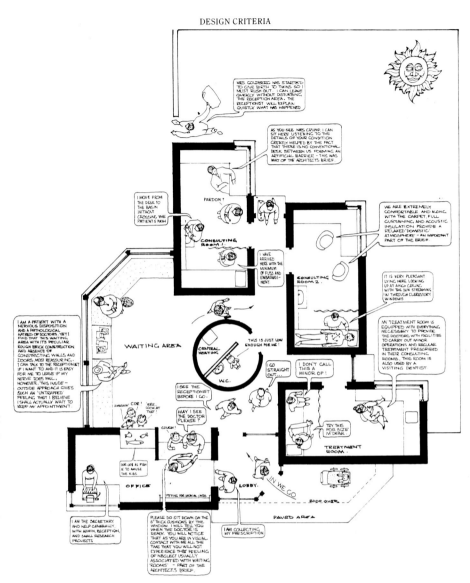

DESIGN CRITERIA

Zoning and patient flow – key points

1 Patients should be able to enter and leave the building without having to walk through a waiting room. Approximately 30% of all visitors will report to the reception to make a general enquiry or to deliver or collect a document and then leave the building. They will therefore not want to wander across the waiting area.

2 The waiting area should have discreet access to a patient WC. This can double as a specimen WC for the treatment area (page 19). As patients' territory, staff should not need to pass through the waiting area. Possible use for group sessions should also be allowed for out of hours.

3 From the waiting area patients circulate into the joint-use territory.

△ *The architects, Aldington Craig & Collinge, encapsulated many of the complex and critical relationships within an illustrative 'working drawing' for their project at Chinnor in Oxfordshire, UK. A refreshing approach to the concept of buildings in use. Illustrations: Aldington Craig & Collinge.*

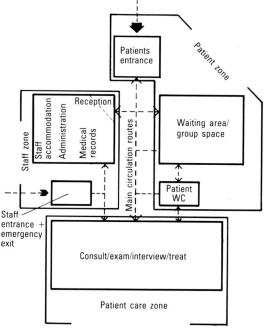

▷ The conceptual criteria for the relationship between the three territories of staff, public and patient care. Larger centres may have more entrances and waiting areas, however the concept remains the same.

4 After the session, a patient may either transfer to another joint-use room (i.e. from consultation to treatment) or leave the building. By passing reception upon exit, a patient will have the opportunity to make, if necessary, another appointment. Note, the patient does not have to walk through the waiting area to leave the building. In cases of emergency (e.g. a distressed patient) it should also be possible for the patient to leave the building via an alternative exit.

5 It must be possible for staff to circulate between staff and patient care territories without having to intrude upon the public spaces. Thus a doctor should be able to enter a building, check in to the records area and then gain access to his consulting room without having to be delayed on route by, for example, a patient in the waiting area.

6 Similarly, staff territory needs to be protected. There will be no need for patients to pass through the staff areas during normal procedures.

7 Flexibility of use. While future change is inevitable, it is often unpredictable. The fact that the building can physically expand will, of course, provide a useful resource for future change. However, because sites are often restricted it cannot be assumed that each centre will have the luxury of an expansion zone. The possibility of change within the building therefore becomes

critical. This does not necessarily imply the ability to relocate positions of partitions, but rather the building's ability to flex to alternative patterns of use and utilization. As previously discussed, if rooms within the building (particularly those involving one-to-one patient care) are of an approximately similar size, such rooms will be less prone to being anchored to one particular function. Functions can change from consultation to examination to interview, etc., without the need for physical or structural alteration within the building (see Chapter 5).

The building environment as a participant in primary health care

An activity-led design can elevate the role of the environment from that of passive container of spaces towards that of an active facilitator of the centre's activities. As such, architecture can at best contribute to the creation of a therapeutic environment, from which an effective and efficient primary health care service can be delivered.

I believe that at best the building itself should have some therapeutic quality
Stephen Gage

References

1. Cammock, R. (1975) Confidentiality in health centres & group practices – the implications for design. *Journal of Architectural Research*, **4**(1), February, pp. 12–13.

2. Filer, G. (1990) Surgery design. *Doctor Magazine*, 4th October, p. 35.

3. Baum, A. and Valins, S. (1977) *Architecture and Social Behavior*. Lawrence Erlbaum Associates, New Jersey, USA.

4. Malkin, J. (1982) *The Design of Medical & Dental Facilities*. Van Nostrand Reinhold, New York, p. 34.

5. Cammock, R. (1977) *Utilization of Consulting Suites in Health Centres*. Medical Architecture Research Unit, London.

6. Cammock, R. (1981) *Primary Health Care Buildings*. Architectural Press, London, p. 66.

The United States of America

Population 1990:	**248.43 million**
Percentage of population aged 65 plus:	**12.2**
Population estimated 2020:	**304.36 million**
Percentage of population aged 65 plus (2020):	**15.4**
Health care expenditure expressed as pounds per person:	**1252**
Health care expenditure expressed as percentage of GNP:	**11.1**

(Source: compendium of Health Statistics, Office of Health Economics, London, UK)

The United States spends far more than any comparable country on health care, yet this is more a reflection of the nation's reliance upon the private sector to deliver a health service to its people. In Great Britain and Scandinavia approximately 90% of health care is financed by central or local government. In the United States public funding accounts for only 40%. There are two public sector programmes – Medicare for the elderly and Medicaid for low-income families, which covers approximately 20% of the population. For the remaining 80% it is simply assumed that people will enter the private health insurance market and purchase their own health delivery system. In practice the main purchasers of health insurance are employers who are able to provide cover for their employees as a tax deductible expense.

However, approximately 13% (34 million) of the population are without any health insurance. This is because only the larger corporations are able to provide insurance for their employees; those employed in small companies, and many self-employed, find it difficult to afford even a rudimentary health insurance cover.

Primary health care is delivered via a diverse range of organizations and building types.

Hospital-based
One form that this can take is as out-patient services delivered by the institution to a strictly out-patient population. The hospital devotes a certain amount of its area to physicians' offices, examination and treatment rooms and the basic ancillary services that would be necessary to support these activities. This would include a small laboratory, a blood-testing station and perhaps a radiology room. It would also draw upon the hospital facility for more complex needs. Almost all hospitals have this type of out-patient activity. In addition, hospitals have tended to co-ordinate with physicians in the supply of land and even building of a medical centre. These would be owned by the hospital and space would be rented by doctors to conduct their private practice.

Health Maintenance Organization (HMO)
HMOs are organized health care systems responsible for both the finance and delivery of a wide range of health care services to an enrolled patient population based upon a pre-paid fixed fee. They are therefore both health insurers and health care providers. HMOs provide health care services to their members through contracts with health care providers on a pre-paid basis.

There are basically four common models of HMO as follows[1]:

Staff model
The HMO builds a medical facility and then directly employs both medical and administrative staff to provide a comprehensive service. The physicians are therefore employees of the HMO.

Group
An HMO forms a contract with one independent group practice to provide health care services.

Network
The HMO forms a contract with two or more independent group practices.

In each case the HMO may still provide the premises, but the medical staff are under a service contract and therefore not directly employed by the

HMO. The HMO may also, however, enter into agreement with a medical group practice which may already have its own premises.

Independent Private Association (IPA)
Here the HMO contracts individual physicians, either single practitioners or a cluster of physicians in the same practice. This has the advantage of low capital expenditure for the HMO. Doctors are paid a fixed fee per enrolment (a capitation) but may also be paid on a modified fee-for-service basis.

The Group Health Association of America Inc., Washington DC HMO factsheet dated August 1990, stated that there were 591 HMOs serving 34.7 million people nationwide at the end of 1989.[2] The HMOs now in operation represent 61 staff model plans, 80 group model plans, 89 networks and 361 IPAs. HMOs provide coverage for approximately 14% of the United States population. Findings from a number of recent employer surveys indicate that HMOs are considerably more likely to cover preventive services in their benefit packages than are indemnity plans.

The concept of the HMO evolved therefore as an alternative to the more traditional systems where an individual who sought health insurance would be a member of an organization such as the Blue Cross or Blue Shield. Costs were rising to such an extent that there was an opening for an organization that could attempt to deliver adequate health services at a much lower price. During the 1980s HMOs have rapidly grown as a major provider of primary health care services, although both Blue Cross and Blue Shield now have established their own forms of HMOs. Operating costs and increased competition, however, leave such organizations vulnerable to the forces of market economics.

Other forms of cover have recently included Preferred Provider Organizations (PPOs). These are insurance plans which offer lower premiums by negotiating a bulk fee for service discounted with particular doctors and hospitals.

In terms of economic viability the minimum size of a primary health care centre in the United States is approximately 500 sq m (6000 sq ft). Sizes however range up to 11,000 sq m (120,000 sq ft) which would be typified by large, independent out-patient facilities.

Typical sizes however range between 1100 sq m (12,000 sq ft) and 2800 sq m (30,000 sq ft) depending upon location and population catchment area.

A further economic factor that is emerging is the delivery of specialized services. While primary services are handled adequately, once a patient requires hospitalization or specialized treatment or diagnosis, such facilities can only be obtained outside the HMO network. HMOs need to contract with local hospitals. Because such specialized treatment is often expensive this can prove prohibitive in terms of insurance costs for the HMOs, if they are not able to contain such services within their own primary health care facilities.

In response to this HMOs are beginning to create speciality centres to avoid dependence on hospitals.

There is also a growing need in the United States for facilities that can treat specific conditions that do not respond well to a hospital environment, for example the Renfrew Center for the treatment of anorexia nervosa (page 68). Such facilities are an important and future trend in primary health care facilities.

As with any commercial building programme, the architecture of primary health care centres will tend to be shaped by how quickly a facility can be brought into operation. This often results in HMOs working with developers who may already own a building shell which would then be fitted out for use as a health centre. This creates complications because a typical developer's building shell may not have the utilities and plan compatible with a preferable medical layout. This inevitably leads to compromises.

In addition to the hospital and HMO medical facilities, there are a large number of small medical centres that have been developed by groups of physicians. These tend to be rented spaces where a physician or group of physicians simply rent accommodation in a commercial building. On occasion physicians will elect to build their own premises as standalone buildings.

Apart from medical centres for physicians there are also surgeon's centres. These are basically an out-patient facility with full operating room capacity not unlike the physician's clinics of Japan.

All of the above building types are set to play a greater role in caring for the nation's future health. Escalating costs of health insurance have brought general recognition for the need to provide a more equitable health service. A shift from surgery to primary and preventive health care is actively being encouraged by Washington as a means of bringing down health expenditure and creating greater opportunities for a more affordable health service.

References

1. The National Health Lawyers Association (1988) A Managed Care Primer: An Overview of the Organization, Operation & Financing of HMO and PPO Plans. (Based upon conference papers delivered by Jerry Coe, Washington Health Network). Alan Gnessin (Alan M. Gnessin), Art Lerner (Michaels Wishner).

2. Group Health Association of America Inc., 1129 20th Street N.W. Washington DC, USA. HMO Factsheet 1990.

3. Robinson, R. (1990) Competition & Health Care: A Comparative Analysis of UK Plans and US Experience, Kings Fund Institute, London.

4. Enthoven, A. (1978) Consumer choice for health plan part 1. New England Journal of Medicine, 298(12), 650–8.

The Valley Forge Health Center

Location:	**King of Prussia, Pennsylvania**
Completed:	**1984**
Type of facility:	**Primary Health Care HMO Health Center**
Architect:	**Wallace Roberts & Todd**
Client:	**The Philadelphia Health Plan**
Gross floor area:	**1020 sq m (11,000 sq ft)**
Photography:	**Tom Crane**

Architect's statement:
Joe J. Jordan, FAIA, Project Design Director

This health care centre comprises an out-patient facility providing primary care and certain specialized medical services to the members of a health maintenance organization (HMO). Subscribers to the HMO pay a fixed annual premium to cover all medical services delivered by the organization. Primary care, including paediatric, obstetric and gynaecological medicine, is offered at the health centre. For more complex diagnoses, treatments and procedures patients are referred to allied hospitals and medical specialists.

The centre is in a developer-built industrial and office park in a rapidly expanding suburban area, King of Prussia, about 30 miles west of Philadelphia. It is located in a single-storey structure with parking and service roads to the north and east and tenant party walls to the south and west. The developer provided the finances for construction of the health centre and passes the costs on to the owner as a monthly rent.

The construction is typical of what is referred to in American as a 'flex building' because its 24 ft high (7.3 m) ceiling permits the flexibility of either light industrial or office occupancy. A structural steel frame supports bar joists and a metal roofing deck while metal studs back up the base brick cladding. Site development and the building shell were designed by the developer's architect, but skylight

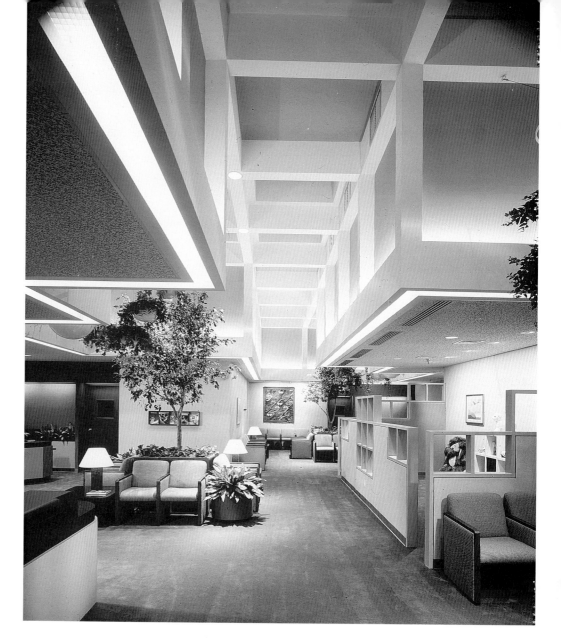

▷ *The Valley Forge*
Health Centre.
Entry/reception.

▽ *Location plan.*

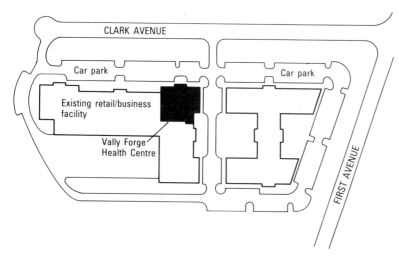

CLARK AVENUE

Car park

Car park

Existing retail/business
facility

Vally Forge
Health Centre

FIRST AVENUE

construction was added as part of the interior
architecture created by WRT.

Of primary importance to the client was a
pleasant and attractive environment for their
patients and a clear and efficient flow of movement
for both patients and medical staff. The visual
impact of the health care centre is an important
marketing consideration to attract new members to
this pre-paid health plan. First impressions are
critical hence the provision of a spacious interior
immediately upon entering the facility, creating
maximum impact.

We planned a visually striking, yet welcoming,
patient waiting area, avoiding the impersonal feeling
of so many crowded clinics. The feel of the space is
quite informal with clusters of seating grouped
around raised planters which are flooded with light
from a system of skylights and illuminated coffers

that burst through the ceiling plane. Another focal
point is the child-scale play space at the centre of
the waiting area. The low step-down partitions with
open 'window frames' permit easy control by
parents and reception staff.

Patients are called from the waiting room by one
of three receptionists, each of whom controls the
entry into a specialized clinical suite. Here the
examination and treatment rooms are grouped
around the nurse work station to enhance visual
supervision by the nursing staff. Within each
medical suite patients and medical staff have
convenient access to a weighing station and toilet,
together with five or six examination rooms and
several consultation rooms.

Variation in finish materials, lighting and ceiling
heights promote boundaries to create clear
differentiation between patient and staff circulation
areas. A continuous service corridor connects all
medical suites with essential supply and
administrative areas, so staff, service and material
deliveries do not have to pass through waiting
areas.

Main waiting areas

Patients
Waiting area (4 × sub-wait)
WCs
Sub-waiting for X-ray
Child play waiting area

Patient care
Examination rooms (× 16)
Eye examination room
Treatment rooms (× 3)
Health education
Psycho-social
Referrals

Staff
Doctors' offices (× 6)
Central reception

Administration office
Manager's office
Staff lounge
Medical records
Central supply
X-ray suite
Janitor's room
Laboratory
Nursing station (× 3)
Eye work station
Staff WCs

Comment

The Valley Forge Health Center conforms to the
functional requirements of a typical medical
practice, yet is within the existing shell of a
developer's building. As a conversion, the deep
plan form is not ideal, with each room competing for
natural light at the perimeter. The deep space also
brings with it the heavier service demands of
artificial lighting, ventilation and cooling. Yet these
plan forms are typical of developers' speculative
building shells in the United States and as a result
the architects paid particular attention to the
lighting design to compensate for the common
absence of natural light.

The deep plan form is also a greater consumer of
energy. As costs escalate more energy efficient
facilities that rely more upon natural daylight and
ventilation will no doubt be favoured.

From entry a patient reports to the central
reception and is then directed to one of the sub-
waiting reception points, each with its own waiting
area. At base level most medical centres tend to
comprise a large number of small rooms linked by a
common system. The architects, however, where
possible attempted to break out of that rigidity to
create instead a series of more intimate spaces
centred around the central sub-waiting areas.
Therefore patients do not have to experience the
whole of the building.

The sub-waiting areas correspond to the different
medical services being conducted within the centre.

▷ *Ground-floor plan*

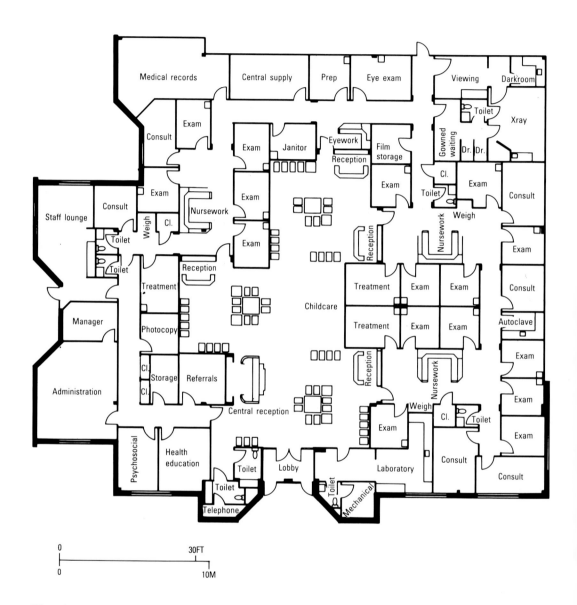

Medical records Central supply Prep Eye exam Viewing Darkroom

Toilet

Consult Exam Exam Janitor Eyework Film storage Xray

Reception Gowned waiting Dr. Dr.

Staff lounge Consult Exam Nursework Exam Eyework Exam Cl. Exam Consult

Weigh Cl. Reception Toilet Weigh

Toilet Exam Nursework

Toilet Reception Nursework Exam

Treatment Consult

Manager Photocopy Childcare Treatment Exam Exam

Treatment Exam Exam Autoclave

Cl. Storage Referrals Reception Exam

Administration Cl. Nursework

Central reception Weigh Cl. Toilet Exam

Psychosocial Health education Toilet Lobby Laboratory Exam Exam

Toilet Exam Consult Consult

Telephone Toilet Mechanical

0   30FT

0   10M

These include:

- General family practice
- Obstetrics and gynaecology
- Paediatrics
- Ophthalmology

After being called from the sub-waiting area patients pass into the respective patient care zones. Each zone comprises a cluster of examination rooms, a doctor's office and a nursing station. Patients are normally shown directly to an examination room by the nurse who supervises and manages the cluster of examination rooms from the nurses' station. If necessary, the nurse will take some preliminary details and prepare the patient for the doctor.

Doctors use their offices primarily as a base and move from examination room to examination room to see their patients. After the examination room

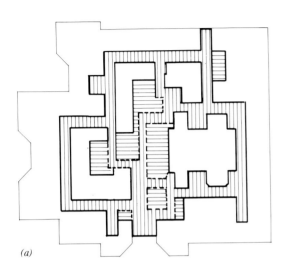

(a)

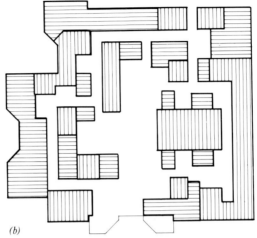

(b)

◁ (a) Circulation and
waiting areas.
▥ Circulation areas.
▤ Waiting areas.

◁ (b) Main functional
areas.
▤ Staff areas.
▥ Patient care.

procedures, patients usually dress and leave the centre.

On occasion the doctor may want to transfer for an X-ray or to undertake an interview/consultation within the more personalized setting of his office.

The Valley Forge Health Center has a clear definition of staff and patient areas, allowing staff to circulate without having to enter the waiting areas.

The clarity of the plan is combined with a concerted approach to good quality lighting, interior design and planting.

Despite having to work within the constraints of an existing building shell, functional requirements of patients and staff are efficiently and skilfully planned within an environment that manages to avoid any

sense of institution.

It is also interesting to note that the Valley Forge Health Center is an example of how the staff/patient flow pattern in United States health centres differs from the United Kingdom model. Patients and medical practitioners will tend to come together in the examination room. Such rooms may not be the exclusive territory of any one doctor and therefore they tend to be less personalized than the doctors' consulting rooms. In the United States the doctor will be on the move, seeing each patient in a different examination room. In the United Kingdom the doctor will tend to remain in his room, which in many cases also acts as his consulting room, examination room and office.

▽ Cross-section.

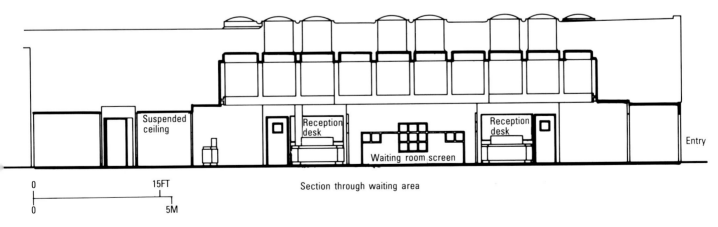

Section through waiting area

0   15FT

0   5M

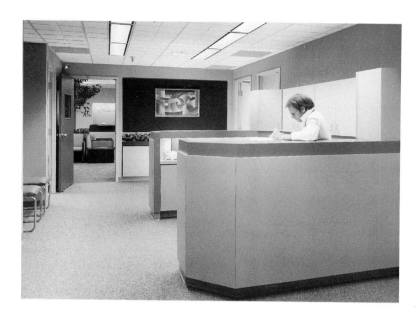

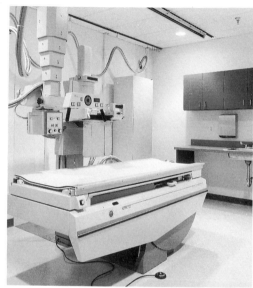

△ *(Left) Typical nursing station.*

△ *(Right) X-ray room.*

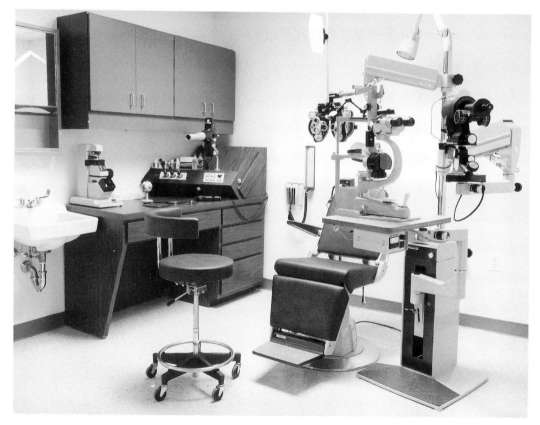

▷ *Eye examination room.*

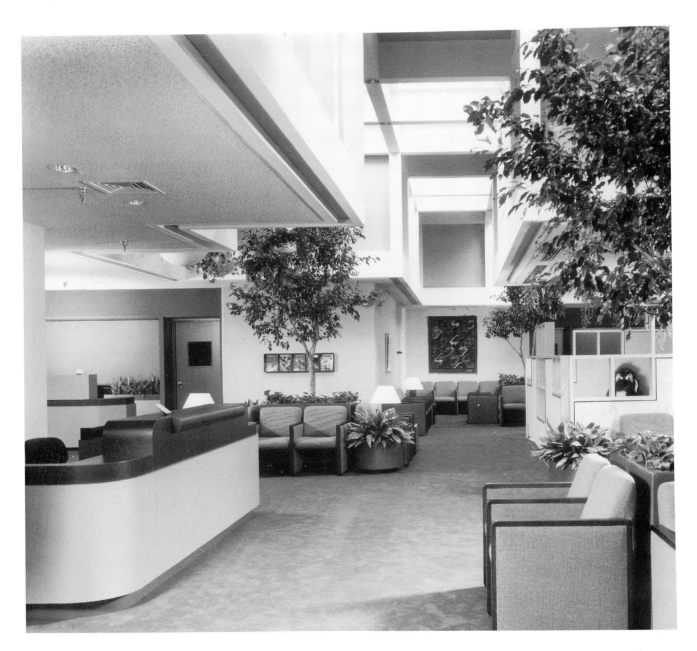

The role of the nurse is also of interest. In the United Kingdom patients tend to visit the nurse for treatment sessions and view the treatment room as her territory. In the United States the nurse appears to follow the role (as in a hospital) of assisting the doctor directly in preparing the patient for examination rather than undertaking certain treatments herself. However, it also has to be stated that the role of the nurse practitioner is now emerging in the United States. The importance of the nurse as a vital member of the primary health care team is increasingly becoming recognized.

△ *Central reception.*

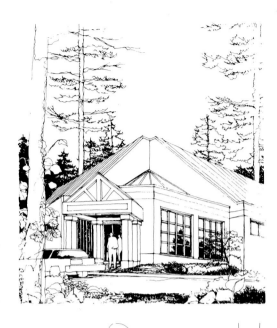

▷ *The Shore Memorial Hospital Ambulatory Care Center. View to entrance.*

▽ *Location plan. The care centre is part of a comprehensive development which includes a medical park campus.*

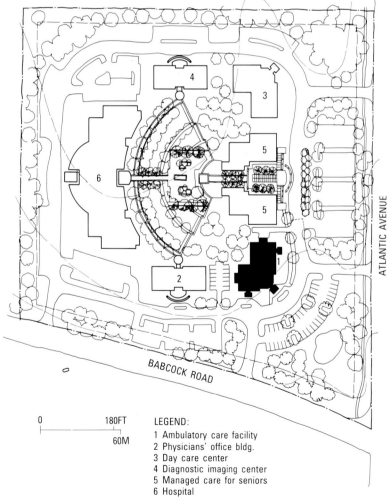

ATLANTIC AVENUE

BABCOCK ROAD

0 — 180FT
60M

LEGEND:
1 Ambulatory care facility
2 Physicians' office bldg.
3 Day care center
4 Diagnostic imaging center
5 Managed care for seniors
6 Hospital

Shore Memorial Hospital Ambulatory Care Center

Location: **Hamilton Township, New Jersey**
Completed: **1992**
Type of facility: **Physicians' care centre with treatment and multiple medical disciplines for related ancillary treatment services**
Architect: **Robert D. Lynn Associates**
Client: **Shore Memorial Hospital**
Gross floor area: **910 sq m (9800 sq ft)**

Architect's statement:
Joseph G. McCaffrey, Project Architect, Robert D. Lynn Associates

Shore Memorial Hospital selected a 20 acre site 15 miles from their hospital in order to develop a free-standing, ambulatory care centre. The master plan for the site includes the future addition of other medically-related components including an Urgi-Care Center* (24 hour operation), a physicians' office building, a physical therapy centre, laboratory centre, medical park for related health businesses and the possibility of a skilled nursing facility.

In order to develop a clear programme which would be understandable to the large number of people involved in the development of the project, we utilized a flow diagram technique to ensure that all parties understood the functional and organizational goals of the programme before a physical design was attempted.

For the first phase of development, the ambulatory care centre, we focused on a physician's diagnostic and treatment suite supporting multiple medical disciplines with provision for related ancillary treatment facilities, including radiology, physical therapy, laboratory testing, etc. The unit

* Urgi-Care
An independent free-standing facility that may or may not be affiliated with a hospital. It has extended hours, usually between 16 to 24 hours per day. It serves a population that may not have access to a private doctor or may have medical needs not serious enough for an emergency. It is fully staffed, with a lab and some medical equipment. The staff will determine if a patient needs hospitalization and will make the necessary referral. About 50% of the Urgi-Care Centers are private enterprises and the other 50% are affiliated with hospitals.

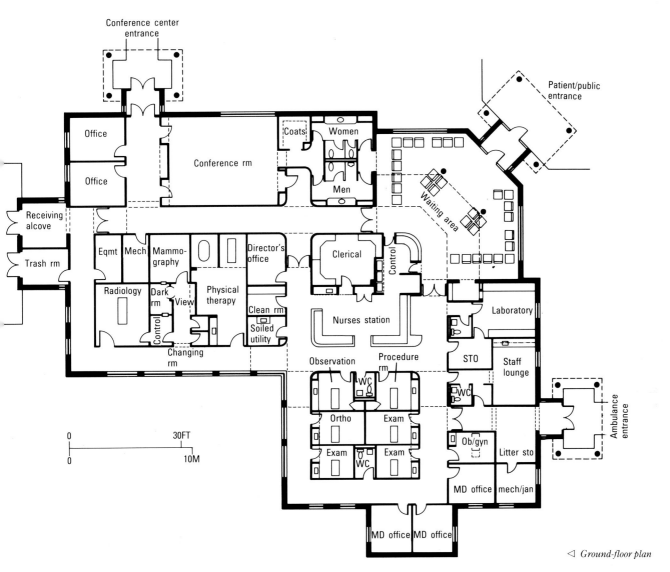

Conference center
entrance

Patient/public
entrance

Office

Office

Coats

Women

Conference rm

Men

Waiting area

Receiving
alcove

Trash rm

Eqmt

Mech

Mammo-
graphy

Director's
office

Clerical

Control

Radiology

Dark
rm

View

Physical
therapy

Clean rm

Soiled
utility

Nurses station

Laboratory

Changing
rm

Observation

Procedure
rm

STO

Staff
lounge

0   30FT

0   10M

WC

Ortho

Exam

WC

Exam

Exam

WC

Ob/gyn

Litter sto

Ambulance
entrance

MD office

mech/jan

MD office MD office

◁ *Ground-floor plan*

is to be supported by public/patient facilities, administration and building support services. In addition, the building will also have to serve as a community conference centre sharing some of the ACC's public support services, but requiring both separate entry and sub-division to permit public use during hours when the medical facility is not in operation.

The goal of the design team was to create a facility which would have clearly understandable

service components with segregated traffic patterns for public arrival, ambulance arrival and delivery/removal services. The facilities were to be arranged to allow for convenient expansion to incorporate major medical components.

The spirit of the architectural design is based upon the desire to create a non-clinical environment with an architectural character that will permit development of future buildings of different scales essentially in harmony with one another.

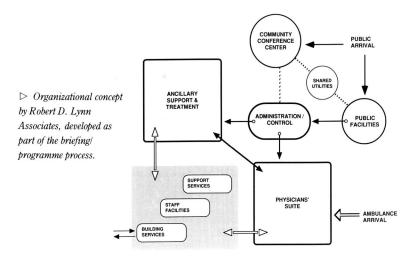

▷ *Organizational concept by Robert D. Lynn Associates, developed as part of the briefing/ programme process.*

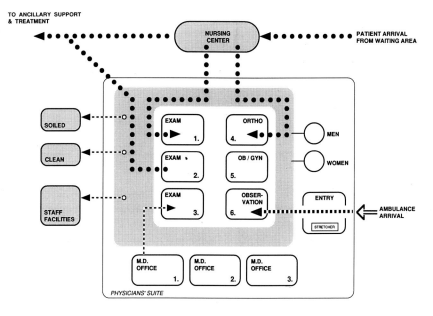

△ *Activity flow diagram by Robert D. Lynn Associates.*

The final design is a one-storey building covering 5 acres of the 20 acre site. The facility will offer primary care, X-ray and diagnostic services, part-time specialists and community educational programmes. It will operate 12 to 16 hours a day, with an emphasis on out-patient services, and is expected to grow with the community's needs. Within a few years of opening, the facility could be capable of offering services in the event of nearby emergencies, such as the stabilizing of trauma victims for transport to a hospital.

The building is designed with three entrances. One is a main entrance directly into the lobby/ waiting area. This will be used during hours when the ambulatory care centre is functioning. Most patients will enter through this main entrance.

Another entrance is located to accommodate public meetings. Educational and wellness programmes can be held throughout the day and after hours. The main lobby can also be used as an additional social space for programmes which warrant this added amenity. Public restrooms are located so that they may be accessed from either the meeting room or the public lobby.

A third entrance is a porte cochere area for the arrival of handicapped patients and the ambulance services which contract with Shore Memorial Hospital.

Main activity areas

Patients
Waiting area
Telephone alcove
WCs
Changing rooms (radiology) ($\times$ 2)

Patient care
Obstetrics and gynaecology examination room
Observation
Procedure room
Orthodontist examination room
Examination room general ($\times$ 3)
Physical therapy
X-ray suite
Conference room

Staff
Office ($\times$ 2)
Clerical room
Control (reception)
Nursing station
Laboratory
Staff lounge
Doctors' offices ($\times$ 3)

Comment

In contrast with the Valley Forge Health Center which stands alone within the community, the Ambulatory Care Center is very much part of an integrated health care complex.

The Shore Memorial Hospital site provides a well co-ordinated series of facilities which benefit from a predetermined site layout. Therefore, each facility can be viewed as part of a whole rather than an after-thought as commonly found on many hospital campuses.

The complex will provide the following:

- The ambulatory care facility
- Physicians' office building
- Day care centre
- Diagnostic imaging centre
- Skilled nursing home

The campus therefore developed the concept of the 'medical park', not dissimilar to the business park or science park where facilities are grouped upon a common site sharing common facilities, each benefiting from the others' presence. As such it can become a one-stop medical facility. The centre is very much identified with the hospital and not with the community, yet within the context of the medical park philosophy its location is valid. It is part of an integrated package of health care services and facilities.

The benefit for both staff and patients will be the ability to draw upon the technical resources and professional expertise of other health care facilities in the park.

The plan follows a rational layout based upon intensive briefing/programme procedures undertaken by the architect. The building has been planned as a series of interrelated zones:

- Community conference centre
- Ancillary support and treatment
- Physicians' suite
- Administration and control

It is interesting to note that the circulation area occupies the perimeter of the south and west areas

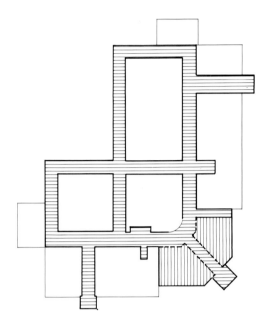

◁ Circulation and waiting areas.

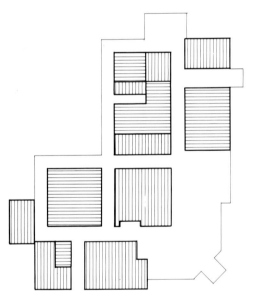

◁ Main functional areas.

of the building. This in turn means that examination rooms are clustered, the position of the corridor forming the favoured 'race track' pattern as found in hospital planning. Apart from the physiotherapy area, none of the ancillary support and treatment rooms would benefit from natural light.

Despite being hospital-based, provision of community groups spaces will allow for health education programmes and bring at least a sense of local community use 'into' the site.

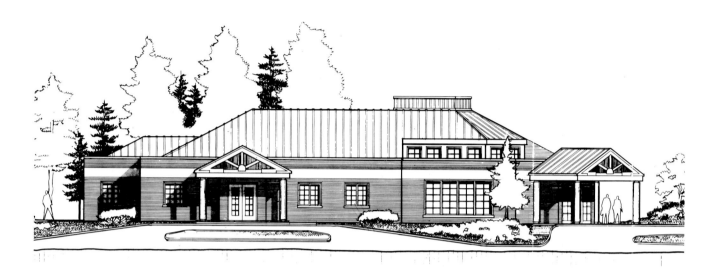

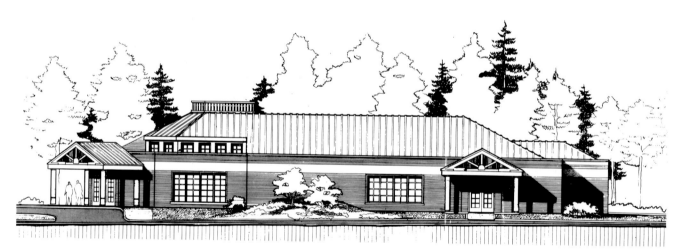

△ *Elevation to Babcock Road.*

△ *Elevation to Atlantic Avenue.*

From entry, patients will report to reception and wait in the waiting space. This is not fragmented as at Valley Forge. From the waiting area patients will pass through into the nursing station area to be shown into an examination room before seeing the doctor. A separate ambulance entrance will give any emergency cases discreet access to or from the building. The same entrance can be used by staff to gain access to their rooms without having to pass through the waiting area.

The centre offers a comprehensive range of health care facilities. Its ability to integrate general medical services, an X-ray suite, physiotherapy and group/conference areas under one roof brings it closer to earlier models of British health centres (page 7). However, its location within a medical park is an interesting and somewhat innovative idea. In the United States the notion of driving to a local shopping mall to buy the week's groceries is now an established pattern. Such patterns are also rapidly developing in the United Kingdom and the rest of Europe. The medical park can be viewed as part of the drive-in-one-stop facility. As such, it opens the debate on location criteria (Chapter 5).

Physicians' Clinic, Myrtue Memorial Hospital

Location: **Harlan, Iowa**
Completed: **1991**
Type of facility: **Out-patient physicians' clinic as part of a comprehensive health care facility at Myrtue Memorial Hospital**
Architect: **Kirkham Michael & Associates**
Client: **Myrtue Memorial Hospital**
Gross floor area: **1279 sq m (13,768 sq ft)**

Architects' statement:
Gary L. Dubas, Project Principal/Designer

Harlan is a progressive mid-sized rural community of approximately 5500 people located in west central Iowa, and is the county seat of Sheby County. From Harlan it is approximately an hour's drive to Omaha, Nebraska, and a one and a half hour's drive to Desmoines.

In the autumn of 1988 the Board of Directors & Administration of Myrtue Memorial Hospital, in conjunction with the various community physicians, collectively decided to embark upon a facility up-grade programme to enhance the quality of health care services offered to the people of Harlan. The goals were three-fold:

1 Consolidate the activities of the three local practising physician groups and that of various regularly visiting specialists into one facility.
2 Expand and improve upon the capabilities and efficiency of the out-patient diagnostic and treatment services, particularly out-patient surgery.
3 Relocate the hospital's main entrance, to function in concert with the new physicians' clinic entrance, thereby offering greater efficiency of visitor and out-patient traffic flow.

These improvements, in combination with services already offered by this existing 52 bed acute care facility, categorizes Myrtue Memorial Hospital as a primary health care centre serving its community and surrounding regions. To satisfy the goals listed above and in order to evaluate and explore the various alternative sites available on or adjacent to the hospital property, an overall site and facility master plan was initially developed. This study included input and the intensive involvement of the Board of Directors, administrative and departmental staff and the area physicians. The advantages and disadvantages of four separate site locations were evaluated, each location involving one- or two-storey options.

From this study the recommended plan of development evolved. The acquisition and development of property immediately adjacent to the south of the current hospital was suggested. This location was considered the most advantageous due to:

- Close proximity and minimal travel distance to/from the current hospital radiology department.
- Excellent vehicular access and high exposure of the main entry to Highway 44 immediately south of this site.
- Good separation of parking and lack of interference with hospital emergency traffic.
- The possibility of hospital expansion to the east.
- An effective functionally-efficient location for a two-level connecting link with the main hospital out-patient and surgery zone, thus separating physician/staff traffic from visitor traffic to and from the hospital.

The proposed project will:

- Relocate the hospital's main entrance, reception and business office zones.
- Add an out-patient pharmacy, gift shop and snack bar near the main entrance.
- Renovate the existing surgery to improve throughput of out-patients.
- The main entrance will also serve the new physicians' clinic.

The clinic will accommodate ten physicians. It will consolidate the medical practices of two family

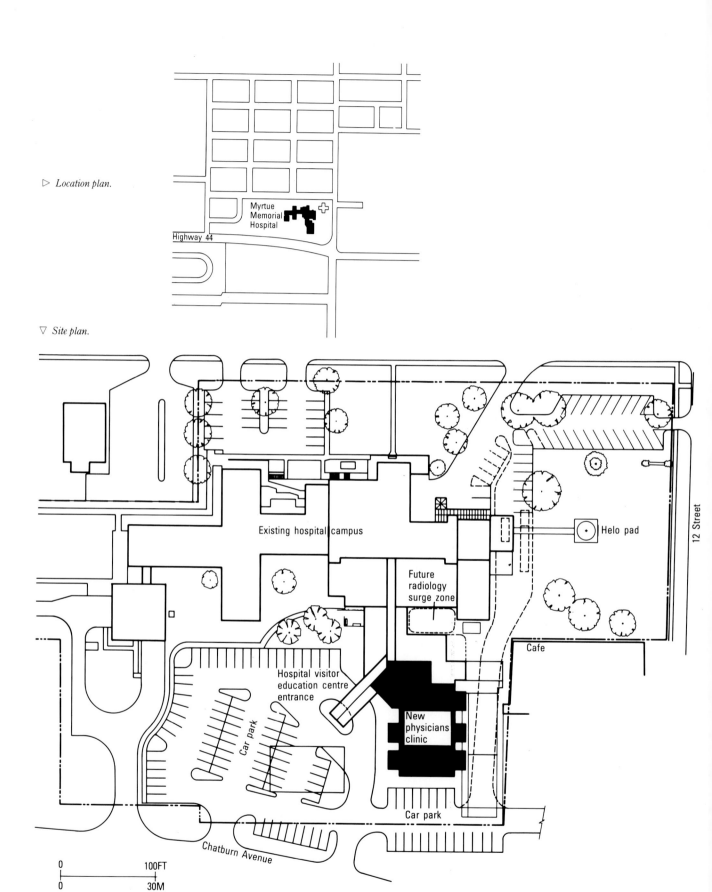

▷ *Location plan.*

Myrtue
Memorial
Hospital

Highway 44

▽ *Site plan.*

Existing hospital campus

Helo pad

12 Street

Future
radiology
surge zone

Cafe

Hospital visitor
education centre
entrance

New
physicians
clinic

Car park

Car park

Chatburn Avenue

0   100FT

0   30M

40

practice physician groupings, a general surgeon and a variety of visiting specialists. The design will easily accommodate a future expansion for two additional physicians.

The design solution was based upon two basic concepts:

1   Optimization of spatial and functional efficiency, through maximum utilization of shared space wherever possible.
2   Establishment of individualized clusters of examination space specific to each practising physician.

The concept of a shared utilization is demonstrated by the multi-purpose common entrance zone, which includes: canopy, Out-patient pharmacy, Snack/vending area, Gift shop, Public toilets.

The hospital radiology department will serve the needs of both the hospital and the clinic. Within the clinic itself, all physicians will utilize one common reception/business office zone and other support spaces such as minor procedures/castroom, laboratory, nurse workroom, lounge, etc.

Individualized clusters of physician activity are created by means of an exam/office module dedicated to each physician. Each module consists of three exam rooms, an office for the physician and a nursing sub-station including charting space, a computer terminal and supply storage. Each module is orientated along the exterior perimeter to allow for windows in all exam rooms and physicians' offices. The windows in the exam rooms have a sill height of 1525 mm (5 ft) for patient privacy.

The facility is constructed in poured concrete footing/foundation systems, steel framework, brick exterior and rubber membrane roofing system. To highlight the main entrance a hip-style sloping roof is included for the front canopy entrance vestibule and main lobby areas. This sloping roof is made of an insulating fibreglass sandwich panel skylight system that allows a high degree of natural light into the spaces.

The exterior of the new addition emulates the colours, textures and detailing of the existing hospital facility. Buff coloured face brick combined with solar grey glass in dark bronze aluminium window-frames is the primary exterior treatment. There are various areas of medium/dark brown brick which reflect the accent, colour and massing of the existing hospital. All brick work includes a variety of horizontal and vertical reveals further to complement the existing detailing.

Main activity areas

Patients
Waiting ($\times$ 2)
Play area ($\times$ 2)
Coats
Telephone alcove
Patient WC
Examination rooms ($\times$ 31)
Minor procedures/cast room ($\times$ 2)

Staff
Doctors' offices ($\times$ 10)
Reception
Medical records
Computer room
Business office
Administration area
Laboratory ($\times$ 2)
Nurse work room ($\times$ 2)
Employee lounge
Nursing sub-station ($\times$ 9)

41

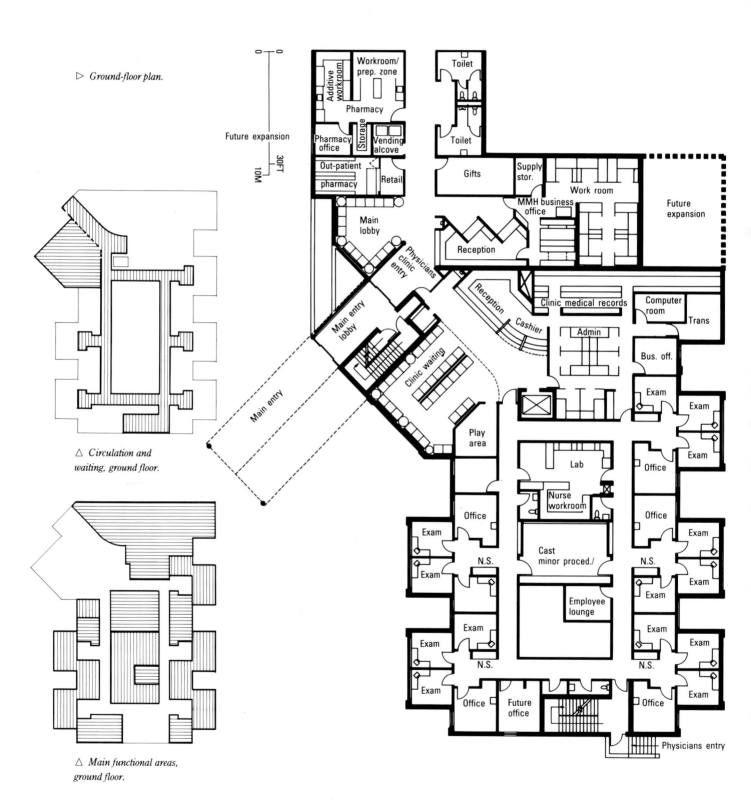

▷ *Ground-floor plan.*

Future expansion

0 ─ 0
30FT
10M

△ *Circulation and waiting, ground floor.*

△ *Main functional areas, ground floor.*

Additive workroom

Workroom/ prep. zone

Pharmacy

Toilet

Toilet

Pharmacy office

Storage

Vending alcove

Out-patient pharmacy

Retail

Gifts

Supply stor.

Work room

Future expansion

MMH business office

Main lobby

Physicians clinic entry

Reception

Clinic medical records

Computer room

Trans

Main entry lobby

Reception

Cashier

Bus. off.

Admin

Main entry

Clinic waiting

Exam

Exam

Play area

Exam

Office

Lab

Office

Nurse workroom

Office

Exam

Exam

Cast minor proced./

N.S.

Exam

Exam

N.S.

Employee lounge

Exam

Exam

N.S.

N.S.

Exam

Exam

Office

Future office

Office

Exam

Physicians entry

42

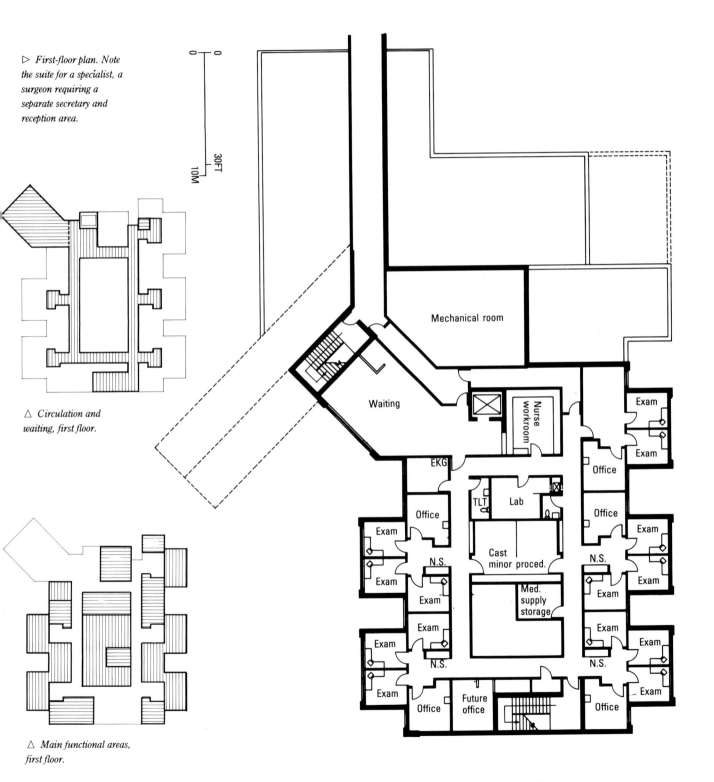

▷ *First-floor plan. Note the suite for a specialist, a surgeon requiring a separate secretary and reception area.*

△ *Circulation and waiting, first floor.*

△ *Main functional areas, first floor.*

0
0
0

30FT
10M

Mechanical room

Waiting

Exam
Exam
Office

EKG
Office
Office
Exam

TLT
Lab
Exam
Exam

Exam
N.S.
Cast minor proced.
N.S.

Exam
Med. supply storage
Exam
Exam

Exam
Exam

Exam
N.S.
N.S.
Exam

Office
Future office
Office
Exam

Nurse workroom

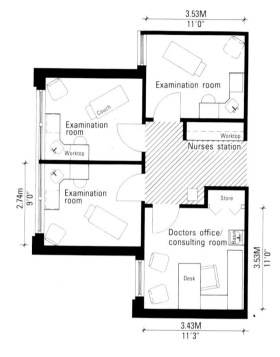

▷ *Typical physician's office/exam suite.*

▽ *Elevations.*

Comment

The Physicians' Clinic is a hospital-sponsored and based facility designed within a similar framework to that at the Ambulatory Care Center at Hamilton Township, New Jersey. Here again its proximity to the hospital is viewed very much as a positive feature, with particular regard to:

- Access to the hospital's technical support facilities.
- Its ease to drive to and park at.
- Having a visible frontage to the main highway.
- Being part of a total health care campus.

In contrast with the Hamilton Township clinic the facility at Myrtue Hospital is physically connected with the hospital at both levels further emphasizing its functional integration with the hospital.

Both hospital and clinic even share a common

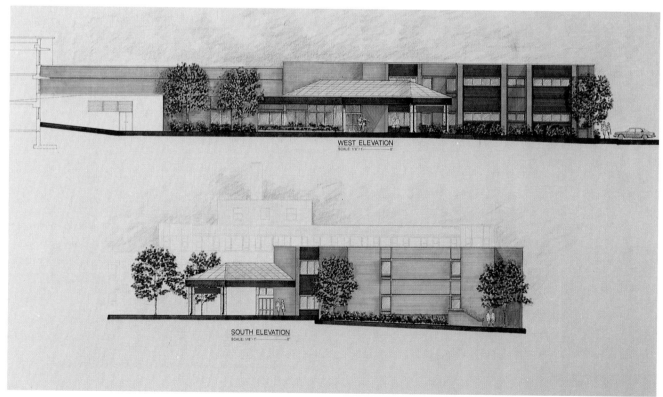

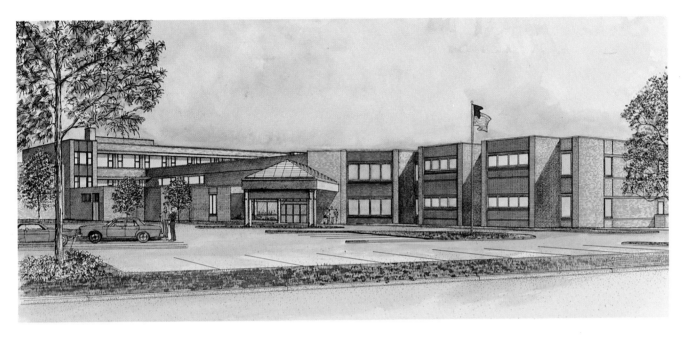

◁ *View to existing entrance area.*

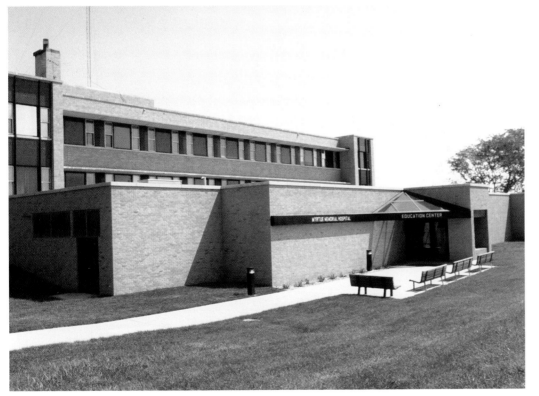

△ *View to proposed new clinic and entrance area.*

45

main entrance. The design for this includes a canopy by the entrance doors allowing visitors to transfer from their cars under shelter. From the main entrance the Physicians' Clinic has a separate sub-entrance. The waiting area is planned within an alcove off the main circulation route, allowing patients to report to reception without having to walk through the waiting room. The waiting area also enjoys a view out on to the main entrance, and can also be visually supervised from the reception point.

At the reception desk the medical records area is screened off from public view. Staff can gain access to the records area without having to cross the waiting area or reception desk.

A staff car park is provided adjacent to a separate staff entrance, thereby also allowing for discreet staff entry/exit to the facility.

The nursing station is expressed as a bay off the physician's office/exam suite with a central nursing workroom on each floor. Future expansion will be possible inside the building shell on both levels; a further six examination rooms and three doctors' offices are allowed for.

The lift is supervised by reception on the ground floor and on the first floor by the nurse workroom which also doubles as a secondary reception point.

Apart from four of the examination rooms planned for the future, all doctors' offices and examination rooms enjoy natural daylight with internal circulation areas. The layout of the physician's suite with a ratio of three examination rooms to one physician follows the American States pattern of functional activity amongst general practitioners in comparison with their European counterparts.

Whilst the merits of the different working methods can only be explained and debated by medical staff, the design results in American centres occupying more space per physician. The combination of consultation, interviewing and examination within essentially one area offers a more efficient utilization of space, although it could be argued that the American model may cause a less efficient through-put of patients.

Kaiser Rockwood Medical Office Complex

Location:	**Portland, Oregon**
Completed:	**1985**
Type of facility:	**Inter-disciplinary physicians' clinic for 36 practitioners providing comprehensive primary health care programmes**
Architect:	**Broome Oringdulph O'Toole Rudolf Boles & Associates BOOR/A Architects Stanley G. Boles, AIA, Principal in Charge**
Client:	**Kaiser Rockwood Medical Office**
Gross floor area:	**4460 sq m (48,000 sq ft)**
Photography:	**Ed Hershberger and Strode Eckert**

Architect's statement:

The building programme was to support 36 practitioners in an inter-disciplinary clinic serving 25,000 patients annually, housed in a facility with the sense of warmth, familiarity and convenience characteristics of a small-scale family practice. In addition to client importance the brief emphasized functional as well as staff efficiency, future expansion and a design that would appeal to the relatively affluent marketplace. Kaiser viewed the project as a prototype for the clinic design and some six future facilities.

As part of Kaiser's regional network of facilities, the project was privately funded through the Kaiser Health Maintenance Organization (HMO), the pre-paid subscription programme of Oregon's largest health care provider. Kaiser currently operates two hospitals and some 20 medical, dental and treatment facilities in its metropolitan Portland area.

With four medical speciality departments this 36 practitioner clinic is organized to achieve adaptable nursing supervision and staffing. Each 16 roomed department surrounds a central nurse station and contains a satellite pharmacy, thus achieving direct visibility and accessibility by nursing staff. Staffing

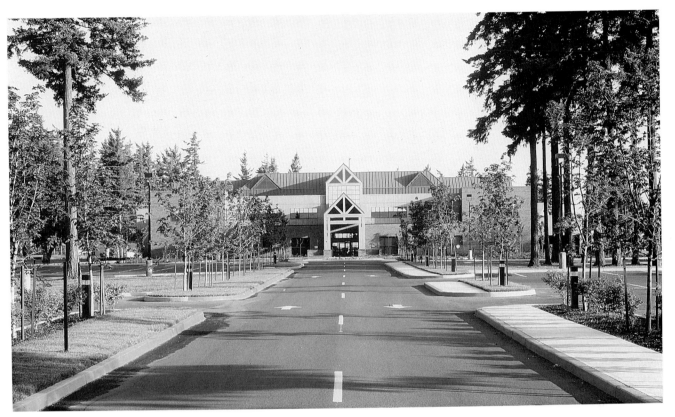

△ *The Kaiser Rockwood Medical Office Complex. View to main entrance.*

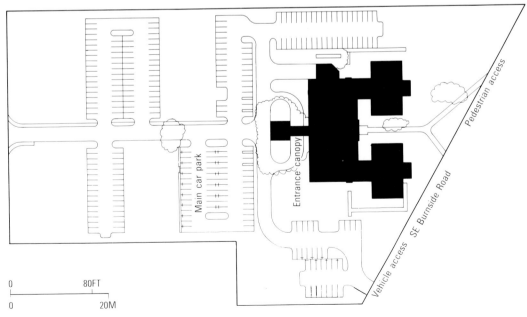

Main car park

Entrance canopy

Pedestrian access

Vehicle access SE Burnside Road

0   80FT

0   20M

◁ *Location plan.*

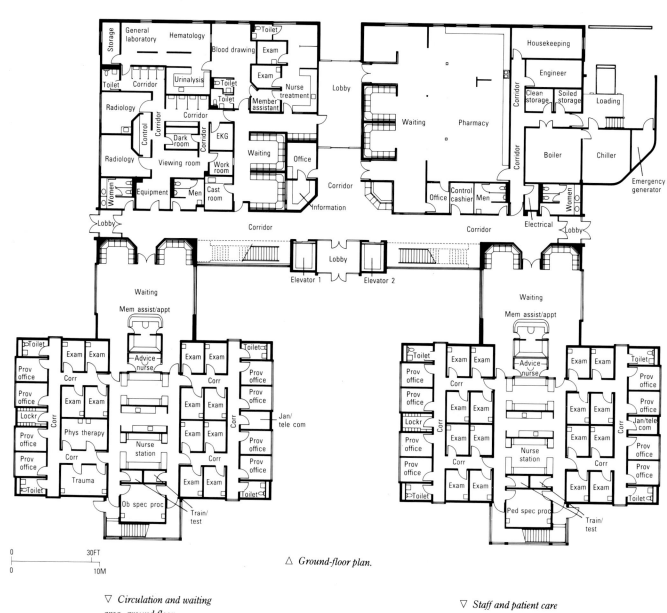

Storage
General laboratory
Hematology
Toilet
Blood drawing
Exam
Exam
Lobby
Housekeeping
Engineer
Toilet
Corridor
Urinalysis
Toilet
Nurse treatment
Waiting
Pharmacy
Corridor
Clean storage
Soiled storage
Loading
Radiology
Control
Corridor
Dark room
Corridor
EKG
Toilet
Toilet
Member assistant
Corridor
Boiler
Chiller
Radiology
Viewing room
Work room
Waiting
Office
Corridor
Emergency generator
Women
Equipment
Men
Cast room
Information
Office
Control cashier
Men
Women
Electrical
Lobby
Corridor
Corridor
Corridor
Lobby

Lobby
Elevator 1
Elevator 2

Waiting
Mem assist/appt

Waiting
Mem assist/appt

Toilet
Exam
Exam
Advice nurse
Exam
Exam
Toilet
Toilet
Exam
Exam
Advice nurse
Exam
Exam
Toilet
Prov office
Corr
Prov office
Prov office
Corr
Prov office
Prov office
Exam
Exam
Exam
Exam
Prov office
Prov office
Exam
Exam
Exam
Exam
Prov office
Lockr
Corr
Phys therapy
Nurse station
Corr
Jan/tele com
Lockr
Corr
Exam
Exam
Nurse station
Corr
Jan/tele com
Prov office
Prov office
Prov office
Exam
Exam
Exam
Exam
Prov office
Prov office
Corr
Corr
Prov office
Prov office
Corr
Corr
Prov office
Prov office
Trauma
Exam
Exam
Prov office
Prov office
Exam
Exam
Prov office
Toilet
Toilet
Toilet
Toilet
Ob spec proc
Train/test
Ped spec proc
Train/test

0   30FT
0   10M

△ Ground-floor plan.

▽ Circulation and waiting area, ground floor.

▽ Staff and patient care areas, ground floor.

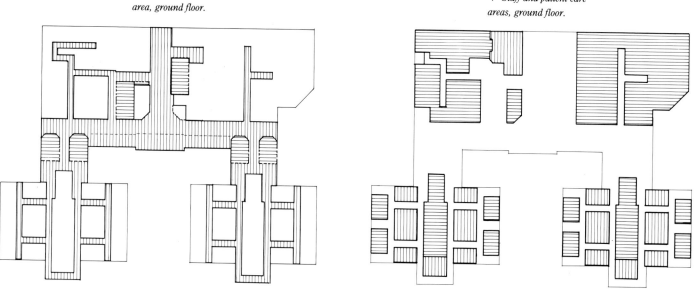

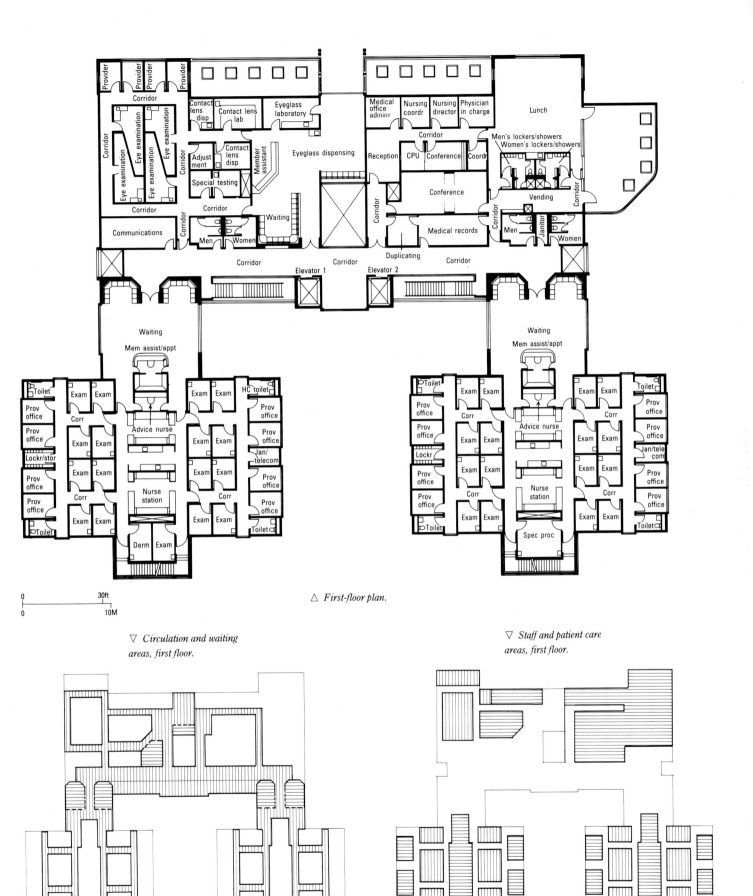

Provider | Provider | Provider | Provider
Corridor

Contact lens disp | Contact lens lab | Eyeglass laboratory

Medical office adminr | Nursing coordr | Nursing director | Physician in charge

Lunch

Corridor

Eye examination | Eye examination | Eye examination

Corridor

Corridor

Adjustment | Contact lens disp

Member assistant

Eyeglass dispensing

Reception | CPU | Conference | Coordr

Men's lockers/showers
Women's lockers/showers

Eye examination | Eye examination

Special testing

Corridor

Conference

Vending

Corridor

Communications

Corridor

Corridor

Men | Women

Waiting

Corridor

Corridor

Medical records

Corridor

Men | Janitor | Women

Corridor | Corridor | Elevator 1 | Corridor | Elevator 2 | Duplicating | Corridor

Waiting

Mem assist/appt

Toilet | Exam | Exam | Exam | Exam | HC toilet

Prov office | Corr | Advice nurse | Prov office

Prov office | Exam | Exam | Exam | Exam | Prov office

Lockr/stor | Jan/telecom

Prov office | Exam | Exam | Nurse station | Exam | Exam | Prov office

Corr | Corr

Prov office | Exam | Exam | Exam | Exam | Prov office

Toilet | Derm | Exam | Toilet

Waiting

Mem assist/appt

Toilet | Exam | Exam | Exam | Exam | Toilet

Prov office | Corr | Advice nurse | Corr | Prov office

Prov office | Exam | Exam | Exam | Exam | Jan/tele com

Lockr

Prov office | Exam | Exam | Nurse station | Exam | Exam | Prov office

Corr | Corr

Prov office | Exam | Exam | Exam | Exam | Prov office

Toilet | Spec proc | Toilet

0 ——— 30ft
0 ——— 10M

△ First-floor plan.

▽ Circulation and waiting areas, first floor.

▽ Staff and patient care areas, first floor.

49

levels are adaptable to each practitioner's change of schedule. Each two level, two department house operates independently. Staff thus assist each patient in the patient's specific treatment setting; there are few reception-only employees.

At the clinic's core the entrance galleria is flanked by a pharmacy, a laboratory, radiology and inoculation areas and leads to a pair of department houses. The resulting village image of smaller, intimate structures is intended to personalize patient and treatment and comfort.

In traditional clinics a 'patient mill' philosophy has existed – impersonal design and institutional autonomy. In contrast Kaiser seeks client and user friendliness in its new facilities.

Kaiser Rockwood's architectural image is intended to promote patient acceptance with its reassuring and warm qualities and also to encourage patients to use the Kaiser system and gain appreciation of its services in comparison with other American health care providers.

The building exterior comprises cedar and brick veneer, lodge-like roofs and red window frame patterns woven into precise, hi-tech yet familiar Pacific NorthWest forms. This ambience of Cascade Mountain lodge forms and geometrically organized materials are carried into the building, where the wood-vaulted circulation route runs from the entrance to the stained, etched-glass window by the artist Ed Carpenter.

Rockwood's main corridor leads to four medical modules stacked as a pair of two-storey houses and a zone for a future additional module. The resulting clinical spaces are personalized by their small size and placement away from central common areas with provision of seating segregated into family obstetrics and gynaecology, paediatrics and internal medicine specialities.

Patient areas have additional features for patient comfort. The areas include small group seating for better choice and privacy, wood lattice ceilings and small aquaria. Glass panels between the seating and nurse working areas foster openness in communication and patient-flow.

BOOR/A held an extended series of project workshops with user groups and representatives. Additional meetings with the Kaiser medical and administrative directors ensured continuity and depth of client involvement, with timely leadership co-ordination during each programme and design phase. Kaiser Permanente (the central HMO client body) performed a post-occupancy study using a questionnaire and survey to evaluate staff and operation efficiency. Staff and patients alike gave high grades to the appearance and operation of the new medical facility. The process of workshops with user groups also led to higher user satisfaction. Those who had participated in the design process identified with the completed project to a greater degree, having been included in earlier discussions.

The clinic provides ambulatory care services in addition to medical specialities for emergency care, minor surgery, optical treatment, radiology, laboratory tests and pharmacy services. The population served lives within 10 miles of the medical facility.

Patients arrive by car at the covered entrance or at nearby on-site parking. They proceed through the front entry via the two-storey access gallery to pharmacy, emergency, optical, laboratory and/or radiology appointments. For speciality care they walk past these general facilities to reach their appropriate medical module. After treatment, patients usually schedule their next visit at the central appointments desk.

The basic structure has concrete foundations, ground slab and wood framing with fire protection by an automatic sprinkler system. Floor materials include carpet and sheet vinyl. Gypsum sheet rock is the basic raw material with wood trim for added warmth in finish. Ceilings are suspended acoustic tile and wood lattice grilles over waiting areas. Mechanical systems are centralized on the main floor area and provide variable volume heated/cooled air ducted to all building areas. Exterior materials include double-glazed windows in painted hollow metal frames, cedar siding and brick veneer. Roofing is painted sheet metal for sloped areas and built up roofing in flat areas.

Main activity areas

Patients

Patient entrance
Waiting areas (sub) (× 5)
Pharmacy waiting
Radiology/inoculation waiting
Physicians' waiting (× 4)
Ophthalmology waiting
Patient WCs

Patient care

Inoculation/laboratory examination rooms (× 2)
Inoculation treatment suite
Physician examination rooms (× 61)
Trauma room
Physiotherapy
Obstetrics special procedures
Paediatrics special procedures
Dermatology room
Special procedures
Eye examination (× 2)
Special eye testing (× 2)
Contact lens dispensing (× 2)
Providers eye consulting room (× 4)

Staff

Physician offices (× 32)
Information desk/office
Pharmacy reception
Physician reception (× 4)
General laboratory/haematology
Blood specimen bay

Laboratory inoculation reception
Radiology room (× 2)
Radiology control
Dark room
Viewing room
Cast room
Work room
EKG room
Pharmacy store
Control cashier
Physicians' nurse station (× 4)
Contact lens laboratory
Eye glass laboratory

Administration

Medical office administrator
Nursing co-ordinator
Nursing director
Physicians in charge
Small conference room
Main conference room
Medical records
Cafeteria
Terrace

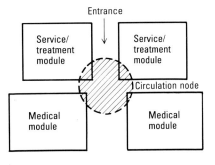

◁ *Planning concept of medical and service treatment modules, providing an economic layout of a multi-disciplinary centre, breaking down the apparent scale for the visitor.*
▽ *Section.*

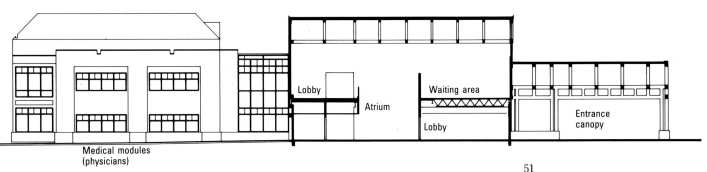

51

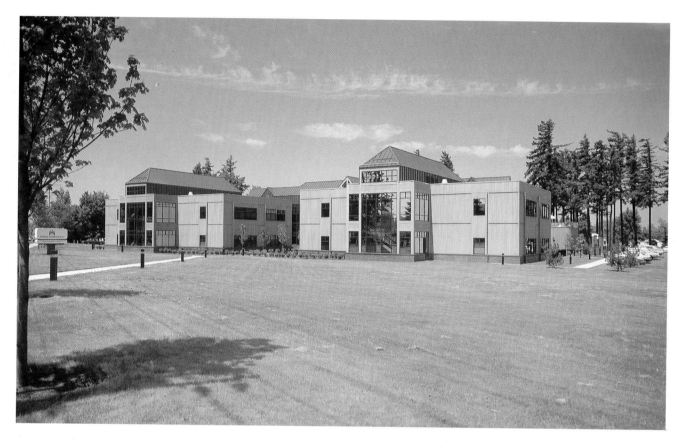

△ *Views from Burnside Road.*

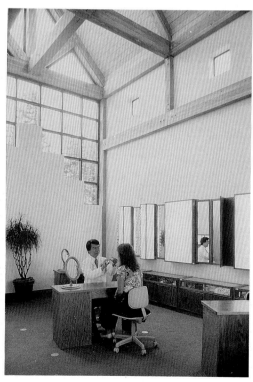

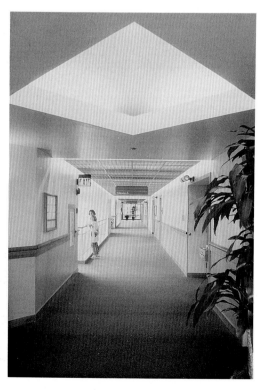

▷ *Typical provider room for optician.*

▷ *Common main floor services are visually open and located close to seating alcoves. A client-orientated layout of the 'medical mall' concept learned from shopping mall design.*

▷ *Open work area of second floor atrium with north facing window wall to glazed side offices.*

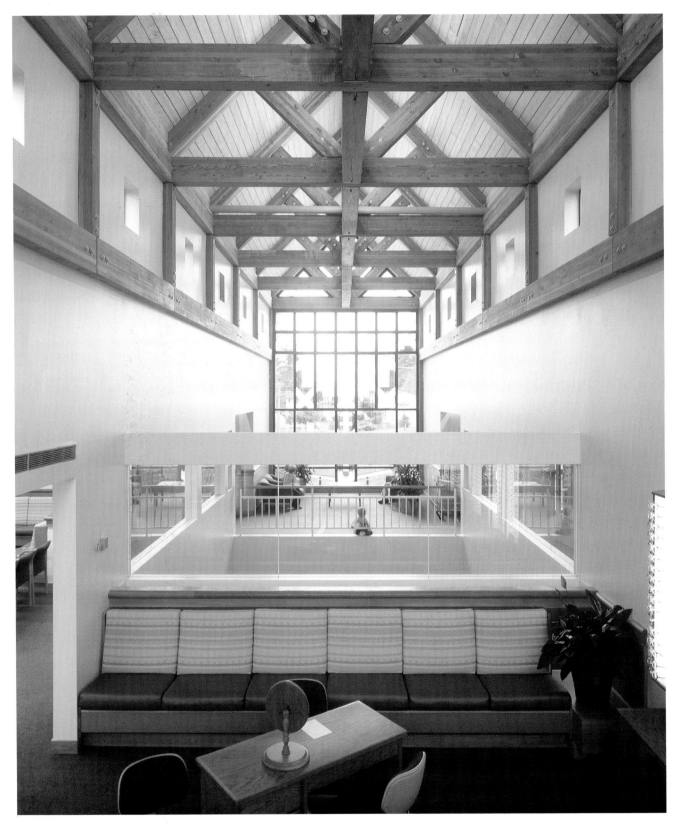

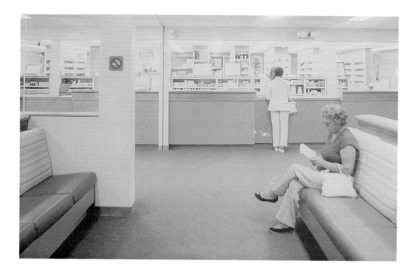

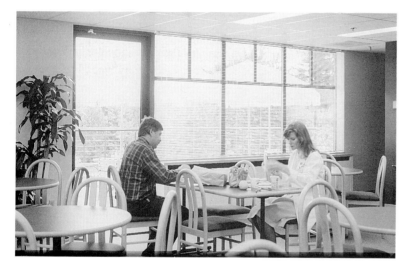

△ *Pharmacy service counter from sub-waiting area.*

△ *Staff cafeteria and outdoor terrace. An unobtrusive method of bringing medical staff together, to encourage opportunities of a primary team approach.*

Comment

Portland has one of the highest physician to population ratios in the United States. As a result, health care is a highly competitive operation. The centre at Rockwood is financed via an HMO programme operated by Kaiser Foundation Medical Care.

The design pays particular attention to the selection of internal materials and finishes which the architects refer to as 'patient friendly'. Despite the size of the facility the concept of separate modules for the various disciplines manages to fragment the scale of the building. Indeed, the reference to a shopping mall seems relevant. The overall structure and support mechanisms of a mall are

large in scale, attracting the shopper to the range of facilities on offer. Yet once inside a particular shop the scale becomes more welcoming and intimate. Such is the experience at Rockwood. The array of medical services under one roof is impressive. The atrium circulation space is large, yet once a patient has located the particular part of the building – or module – in which the consultation or treatment is to take place, the environment changes from one of impressive confidence to a more reassuring intimacy.

Apart from an atmosphere and energy generated by the spaces within the building, the scheme's medical planning embraces functional and economic efficiency. The basic layout of the physicians' clinic area is duplicated four times, one for each discipline. The service modules are then linked via a circulation node. This allows an economy of scale in design and construction, so critical to this type of facility. In developing the standard module the architects worked very closely with their client so that once an optimum layout was generated it could not only be repeated within the proposal, but further modules could be added in future, linking through to the circulation node.

While the layout of the centre allows various medical disciplines to deliver their services within the semi-autonomous modules, the design also incorporates the opportunity for staff integration. For example, the provision of a cafeteria provides an unobtrusive means for social interaction between staff. The centre also has two conference rooms. There is therefore an opportunity for members of staff to work as a team, in concord with the concept of a primary health care building.

The post-evaluation study undertaken by the client revealed a high degree of user satisfaction. This is probably due to the very thorough methods undertaken to determine the brief/programme for the building and the integration within the design of the management and staffing needs. The architects also designed with the market (i.e. the prospective patient) in mind. As the provision of medical buildings moves toward meeting the needs of the consumer and not just the medical consultant, the approach of the architects in designing the Rockwood Center has a place in the debate on medicine and architecture through its recognition of the patient as not necessarily a humble recipient, but as the purchaser of health services with the power of choice.

54

The Straub Mililani Family Health Care Center

Location:	**Mililani, Hawaii**
Completed:	**1988**
Type of Facility:	**Walk-in multi-disciplinary medical clinic including doctors' offices, obstetrics and gynaecology, and paediatrics**
Architects:	**Media Five Ltd**
Client:	**Straub Clinic & Hospital Inc.**
Gross floor area:	**654 sq m (7035 sq ft)**
Photography:	**Ron Star**

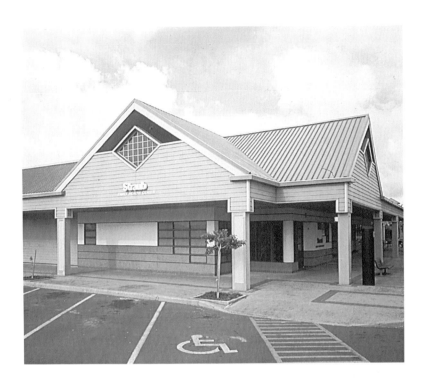

Architect's statement:

The Straub Mililani Family Health Care Center is a walk-in medical clinic located in Mililani town's new shopping centre in Hawaii.

The client, Straub Clinic Hospital Inc., wanted to create a comprehensive neighbourhood clinic which projected a professional yet residential atmosphere. The exterior needed to signal the clinic's presence in the community while complying with the overall visual consistency of the Mililani town centre. In addition, the clinic had to meet or exceed the standards set by the client's already established clinics (in Kailua and Kaneohe, Hawaii). All of these requirements had to be achieved within the guidelines of an economical budget.

Media Five Ltd provided architectural designs for the facade, interior and signage for the project. This included the street/pedestrian mall entrance, examination rooms, X-ray laboratories, obstetrics/gynaecological examination rooms, doctors' offices, conference room, paediatrics area, reception lobby, waiting room with children's play area and nursing station.

The facade integrates the neighbourhood clinic with the setting of the Mililani town centre through a consistent use of colour and materials. Its signage is emphasized clearly to delineate the clinic as a separate business from the parking area. Blue trim work and multi-panelled glass windows framed with wood help to increase its distinction from the shopping area.

The interior was designed to create a pleasant

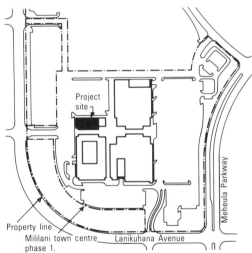

△ *Straub Mililani Family Health Care Center, Mililani, Hawaii, USA. View to main entrance.*

◁ *Location plan. The Health Center is situated within a new shopping centre at Mililani. It enjoys good access to the neighbourhood as a community resource.*

home-like feeling. Indirect lighting and soft colours create a soothing atmosphere. The sculptured mouldings and ceiling help to project the image of a modern, professional office. Blue trim work and wooden grid dividers repeat the details of the building exterior, and help to separate the waiting areas from the reception desk. The children's play area is further defined by frosted glass panels inserted in the wooden grid. The carpeting, finishes and upholstery were selected for their durability and low maintenance needs.

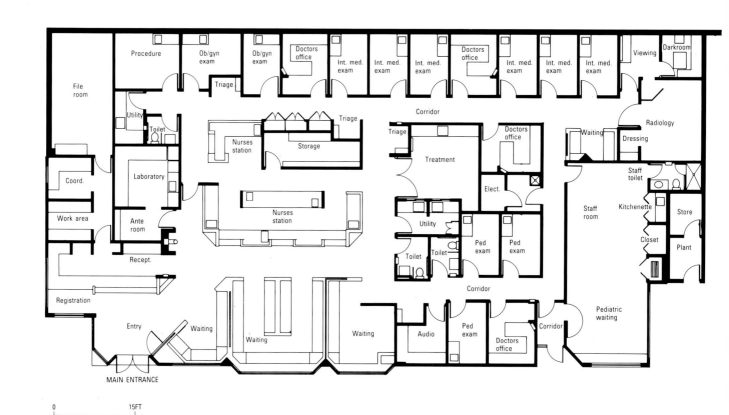

△ Ground-floor plan.
There is accommodation for
a range of family health
services within one
integrated facility.

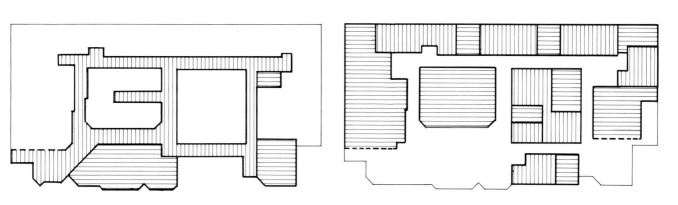

△ Circulation and
waiting.

△ Main functional areas.
Staff and patient care.

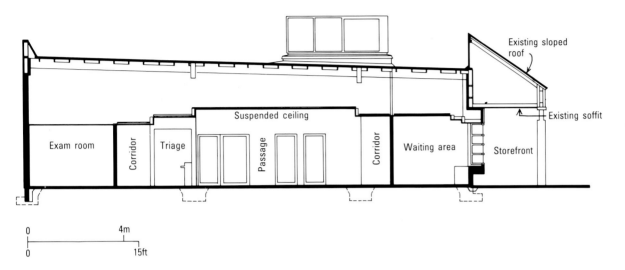

△ Cross-section through the building.

Main activity areas

Patients

Waiting – main wait (sub-divided into three sub-waiting areas)
Paediatric waiting
Internal medicine sub-waiting
Patient WCs

Patient care

Paediatric examination (× 3)
Audio
Radiology dark room
Internal medicine examinations (× 6)
Treatment
Obstetrics and gynaecology examination rooms (× 2)
Procedures room

Staff

Doctors' offices (× 4)
Staff room
Dark room
Radiology viewing
Utility (× 2)
Laboratory room
Nursing stations (× 2)
Reception
Office area
Records room

Comment

The Straub Family Health Center embodies the basic planning concepts of American primary health care design. The main characteristic is the cluster of examination rooms around the doctor's office.

The main entrance works particularly well. The transition from public to private space begins on entering the building under a colonnade. Once at the front entrance door all those who enter and leave the building can be visually supervised. The angle of the reception desk to the main circulation route into the building allows visitors to report to reception without causing disruption to those leaving the building who do not need to see the reception staff again.

The waiting areas are deliberately fragmented to reduce their apparent scale, allowing for a more relaxed area in which to wait for a consultation. From the waiting room patients are directed to any one of the three major examination room zones, i.e. obstetrics, internal medicine or paediatrics.

At the centre of the building are the nurses' station, treatment and utility rooms which, if required, can serve all medical areas.

The paediatric waiting room can also be expanded if necessary, via a folding partition, into the staff room. The allows the opportunity for group sessions in health prevention or other community health programmes.

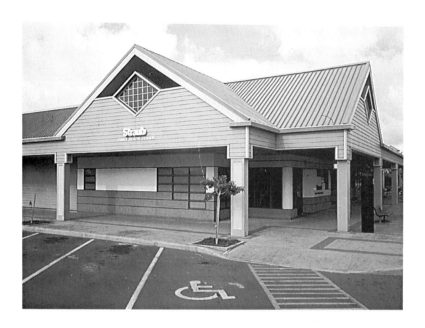

△ *View to main entrance. The centre was constructed around an existing shell, fitted out and a new exterior facade added. Full consideration was given to access for disabled visitors. Note the designated car space and drop kerb in the forefront.*

▷ *Waiting sub-area utilizing graphics to informalize the space, yet providing a relaxing and secure environment for patients awaiting their consultations. Note the magazine rack built into the wall panel offering a tidy solution to the common problem of magazines strewn about a waiting area.*

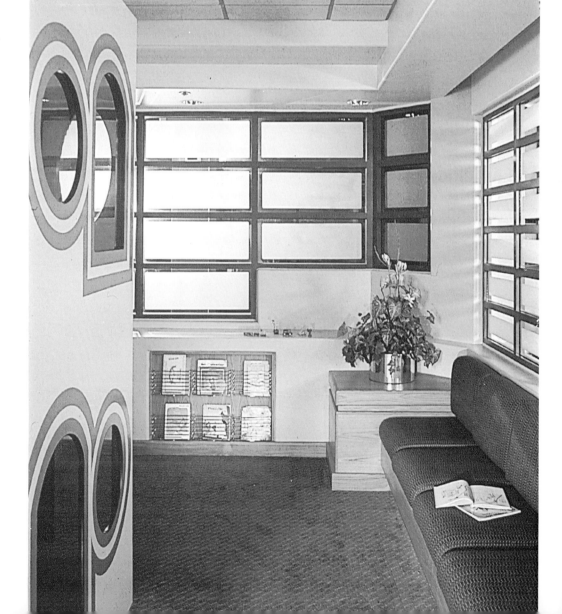

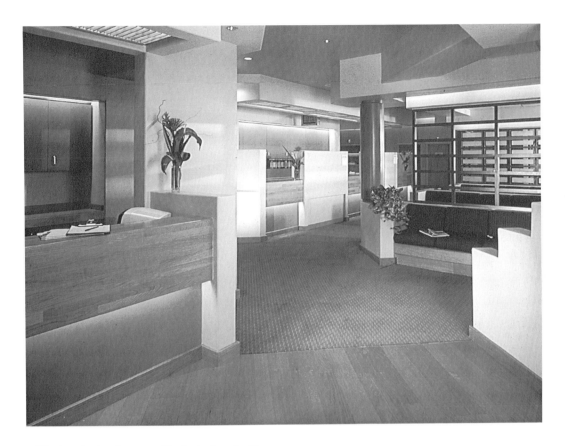

◁ *Views looking towards nursing station with the main reception desk on the left and one of the three front sub-waiting areas to the right.*

▽ *Close-up of nursing station. Media Five, as a multi-disciplinary practice, also integrated signage and other graphics into the design.*

The interior has been sensitively designed with much thought given to the choice and blend of materials and fixtures. The image is that of a well organized, professional office, which avoids a clinical appearance. As a multi-disciplinary practice, the architects have also incorporated signage and other graphics into the design. The interior planning reflects a developing project relationship between Media Five and Straub over a series of health centres, each gaining from a consolidation of experience and a greater understanding of client and user needs through the evaluation of past projects.

As with the Valley Forge Health Center (page 27) the Straub Family Health Center is part of a neighbourhood shopping centre. It is therefore able to command a public profile within the fabric of the local community. As at Valley Forge, visiting the centre does not necessarily require a special journey. It becomes merely part of a routine visit to the shopping centre. Because of its location, health screening and preventive programmes stand a better chance of success in terms of attracting sufficient numbers to attend regular sessions.

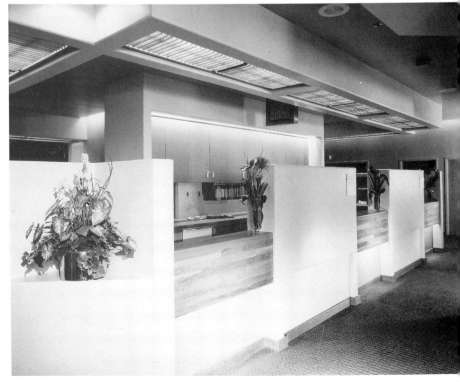

Inscription House Health Center

Location:	**Kayenta, Arizona**
Completed:	**1983**
Type of facility:	**Multi-disciplinary primary care clinic and 24 hour emergency care centre within an American-Indian reservation (prototype facility)**
Architects:	**Drover Welch & Lindlan (DWL) Architects**
Client:	**Navajo Area Indian Health Service, USA Department of Health & Human Services**
Gross floor area:	**1800 sq m (19,480 sq ft)**
Photography:	**Terrance Schlesinger**

Architect's statement:
Carleton W. Van Deman (President of DWL), Principal Designer

Set amidst the shifting dunes and soaring buttes which characterize the high desert plateau of the sprawling Navajo Indian Reservation, the Inscription House Health Center is from a technological standpoint an innovative building, as well as a unique design for a very specialized patient population. This out-patient facility is located on a 54 acres (22 hectare) site in Northern Arizona, at an approximate elevation of 6300 ft (1920 m) where it is subjected to snow and severe cold in winter and temperatures in excess of 100 °F (37 °C) in summer. It serves a population of approximately 5000 Navajo Indians who occupy a sparsely populated region of over 500 square miles (1300 sq km). The Navajo nation is the largest Indian Reservation in the United States encompassing some 25,515 square miles (66,000 sq km) in the western United States. The Navajo Area Indian Health Service, a unit of the United States Public Health Service, is responsible for health care on the reservation. Care is provided by the Government for all Navajos free of charge. Health care services include primary care and

dental care at facilities such as Inscription House, acute in-patient care at hospitals located throughout the reservation, and specialized diagnosis and treatment facilities at the Regional Referral Center in Gallup, New Mexico.

In 1980 when awarded this commission, DWL personnel began extensive research into this special patient population. They investigated tribal traditions, tribal politics, the Navajo heritage and view of the land. Native healing practises were included, and their interface with modern medicine, as well as the issue of services such as distance people travel to receive care. Further research was conducted on the site and dealt with climate, lack of utilities and location of nearest roadways. The information package provided a comprehensive overview of the community and the people being served. For example, a significant proportion of the patient population consisted of elderly Navajos who did not speak English. As a result, DWL's response was to establish a design criteria that would develop a building with simple movement pathways and provide for the utilization of symbols for directional signage rather than language direction graphics.

The Inscription House Center houses a 24 hour

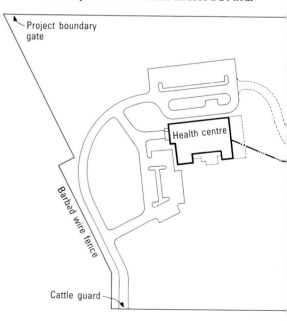

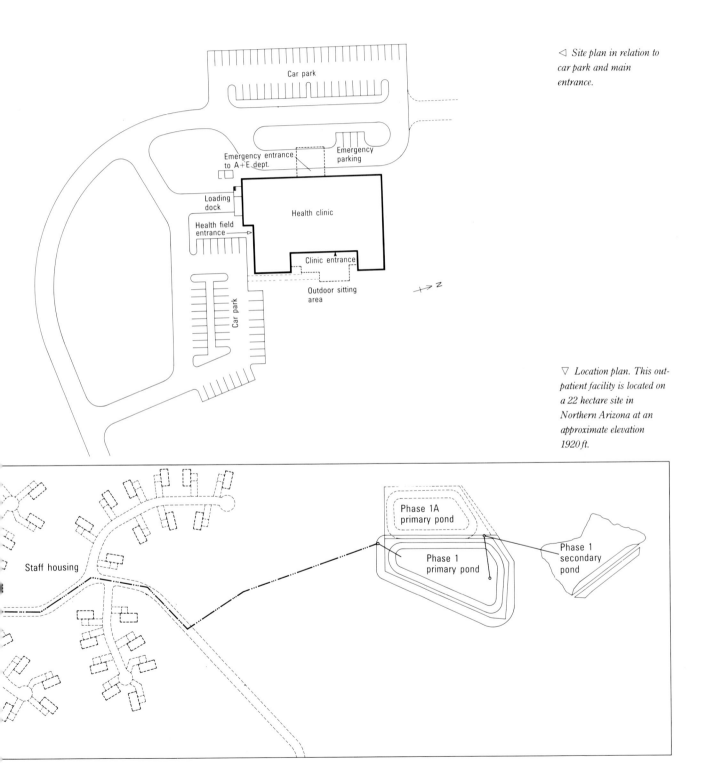

◁ Site plan in relation to car park and main entrance.

Car park

Emergency entrance to A + E dept.

Emergency parking

Loading dock

Health clinic

Health field entrance

Clinic entrance

Car park

Outdoor sitting area

N

▽ Location plan. This out-patient facility is located on a 22 hectare site in Northern Arizona at an approximate elevation 1920 ft.

Phase 1A primary pond

Phase 1 primary pond

Phase 1 secondary pond

Staff housing

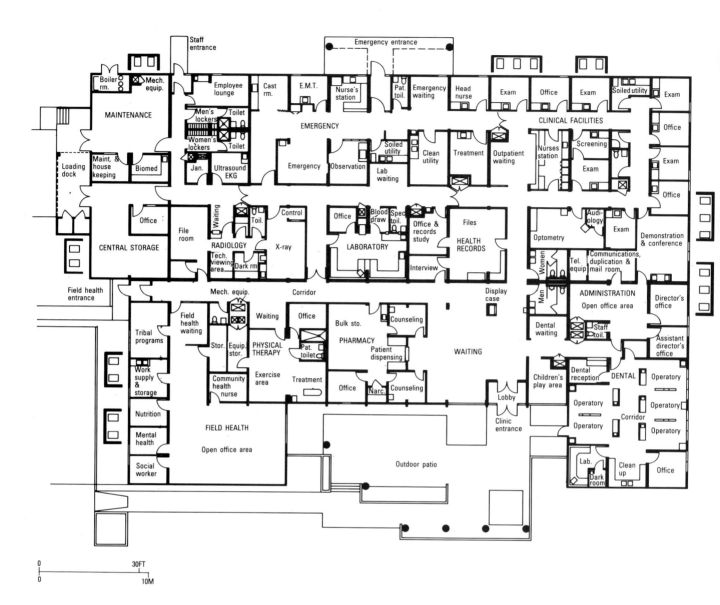

Boiler rm.
Mech. equip.
MAINTENANCE
Staff entrance
Employee lounge
Cast rm.
E.M.T.
Nurse's station
Pat. toil.
Emergency waiting
Head nurse
Exam
Office
Exam
Soiled utility
Exam
CLINICAL FACILITIES
Office
Men's lockers
Toilet
Women's lockers
Toilet
EMERGENCY
Exam
Loading dock
Maint. & house keeping
Biomed
Jan.
Ultrasound EKG
Emergency
Observation
Soiled utility
Clean utility
Treatment
Outpatient waiting
Nurses station
Screening
Office
Lab waiting
Exam
CENTRAL STORAGE
Office
File room
Waiting
Toil.
Control
Office
Blood draw
Spec toil.
Office & records study
Files
HEALTH RECORDS
Audi- ology
Exam
Demonstration & conference
RADIOLOGY
X-ray
LABORATORY
Optometry
Field health entrance
Tech. viewing area
Dark rm
Interview
Women
Tel. equip
Communications, duplication & mail room
Mech. equip.
Corridor
Display case
Men
ADMINISTRATION
Open office area
Director's office
Tribal programs
Field health waiting
Waiting
Office
Bulk sto.
Counseling
Dental waiting
Staff toil.
Assistant director's office
Stor.
Equip. stor.
PHYSICAL THERAPY
Pat. toilet
PHARMACY
Patient dispensing
WAITING
Children's play area
Dental reception
DENTAL
Operatory
Work supply & storage
Exercise area
Treatment
Office
Narc.
Counseling
Lobby
Operatory
Operatory
Community health nurse
Clinic entrance
Corridor
Operatory
Nutrition
FIELD HEALTH
Open office area
Outdoor patio
Operatory
Mental health
Lab.
Clean up
Office
Social worker
Dark room

0   30FT
0   10M

△ *Ground-floor plan.*

emergency care centre, a large out-patient primary care clinic, a dental clinic and a large pharmacy with consultation spaces for teaching the administration of medication. Diagnostic facilities include radiology and a laboratory. The clinic has a physical therapy area and offices for home-help nursing staff and a nutritionist. Primary care and dental clinics are an 8.00am to 5.00pm operation and are zoned close to the building entry with ready access to a patients' records area. The pharmacy is directly accessible to the waiting area and is passed as patients leave the building. Direct access from the exterior to the home-help area is provided so these staff members do not need to traverse the entire building. Radiology and a laboratory are located between emergency and primary care to provide easy access to both. During evening hours when staffing is

limited, two-thirds of the building can be shut down and all remaining functions carried out in the active space.

The exterior of the building is covered with insulated panels of low-maintenance synthetic stucco. The panels have depressed areas where feature strips of ceramic tile are installed. Redwood exterior panelling accents the main building entry. The modular design limited the building's total height to 3.6 m (12 ft). The entry patio is covered with steel shade structures, each of a pyramid shape set on free-standing concrete columns to provide an entry focal point, while in keeping with the Navajo tradition. This tradition is based upon the belief that building entries should face east and be positioned so that major shadows do not obscure the doorway. Exterior fenestration was kept to a

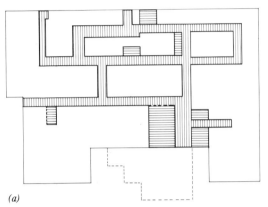

(a)

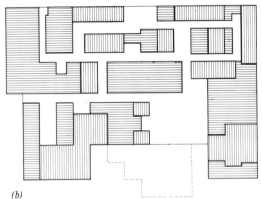

(b)

◁ *(a) Waiting and circulation areas.*

◁ *(b) Staff and patient care areas.*

minimum for energy conservation. All major fenestrations are in the dental area where views are maximized.

The health centre was completely financed by federal funds. It is part of a total complex which includes housing units for residential staff and the traditional Navajo healer's Hogan. Utilities are provided on site with the centre's own water-well and sewage treatment system. The Center promotes the efficient use of Indian Health Service physicians and nurses and contributes to the on-going effort of the United States Government to bring the quality of care on a reservation up to the standard of that of the general population.

The Inscription House Health Center was an experimental project for the United States Indian

Health Service (IHS). As a response to the remote location of many of its facilities, IHS decreed that investigations should be conducted into building clinics in off-site, pre-manufactured modules. Therefore DWL designed the Inscription House Clinic as 28 modules which could be built in an off-site factory, trucked to their final location and assembled. This design criteria was considered along with other remote location factors such as self-sufficiency and ease of maintenance. The heating, ventilating, air-conditioning system for example is very simple and can be maintained by local staff. After careful consideration of cost factors the pre-manufactured construction option was ultimately deferred, and the facility was site-built using wood-frame construction.

▽ *Section. DWL designed the Inscription House Clinic as 28 modules which could be built in an off-site factory, trucked to their final location, and assembled.*

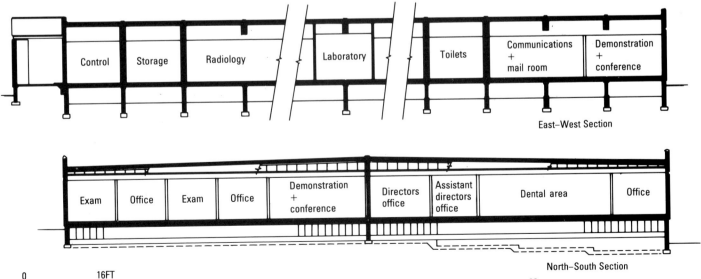

| Control | Storage | Radiology | | Laboratory | | Toilets | Communications + mail room | Demonstration + conference |

East–West Section

| Exam | Office | Exam | Office | Demonstration + conference | Directors office | Assistant directors office | Dental area | Office |

North–South Section

0   16FT

0   5M

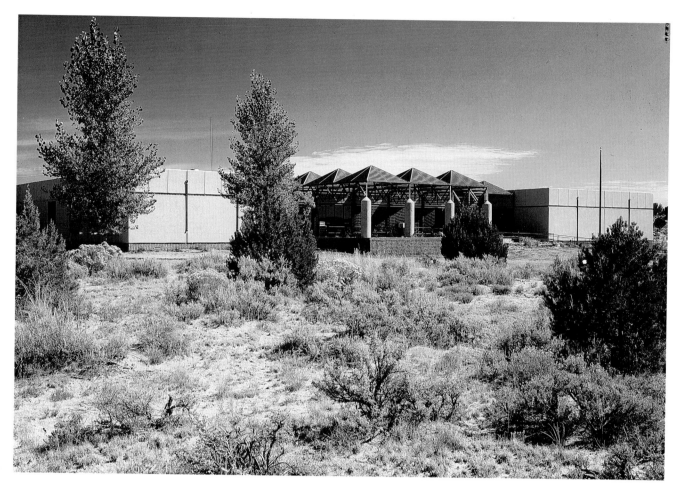

(a)

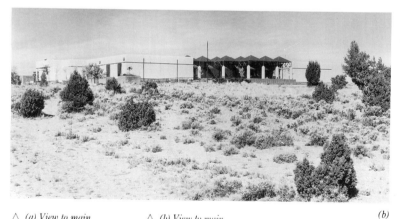

(b)

△ *(a) View to main entrance. The Center is set amidst the shifting dunes and soaring butts which characterize the high desert plateau of the sprawling Navajo-Indian Reservation.*

△ *(b) View to main entrance. The Center is set amidst the shifting dunes and soaring butts which characterize the high desert plateau of the sprawling Navajo-Indian Reservation.*

Main activity areas

Patients
Main waiting
Outdoor patio
Children's play area
Dental waiting
Patient WC
Out-patient waiting
Laboratory waiting
Emergency waiting
Radiology waiting
Physical therapy waiting
Field health waiting

Patient care
Dental operatory bays ($\times$ 5)
Examination rooms (clinics) ($\times$ 6)
Screen room optometry, history and physical

Treatment room
Observation room
Emergency room
Cast room
Ultra-sound room
Demonstration and conference room
X-ray room
Tribal programme room
Consultation room (field health)
• Nutrition
• Mental health
• Social worker
• Community health nurse
Field health group space
Exercise area
Physical therapy – treatment
Counselling room (× 2)

Staff
Open area office
Director's office
Assistant director's office
Dental reception
Dental laboratory
Dentist's office
Dark room
Mail room

Doctors' offices (× 3)
Soiled utility (× 2)
Clean utility
Health records
Main reception
Office and records study
Nursing station (× 2)
Laboratory
Head nurse's office
Radiology dark room
Radiology file room
Central storage
Central storage office
WCs

Maintenance
Maintenance and house keeping office
Employee lounge
Male lockers
Female lockers
Loading dock

Comment

Outside the sphere of private medicine, and largely outside what has become contemporary American culture, lies one of the remaining American-Indian

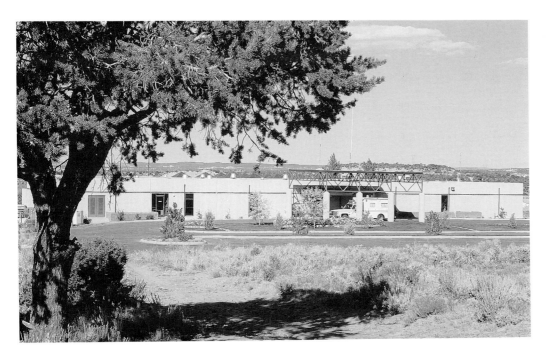

◁ *View of emergency entrance at rear of building. The Center also has separate entrances for field health staff who work in the community, as well as the main entrance which serves the pharmacy, dental clinic and physical therapy facilities.*

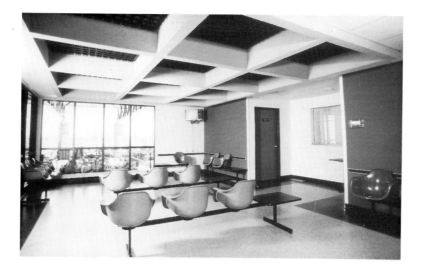

△ Main entrance area looking back to the outdoor patio with one of the counselling rooms to the right.

reservations. Their community of indigenous Americans, the largest reservation in the United States is, however, sparsely populated. Five thousand Navajo Indians inhabit a territory of 500 square miles (1290 sq km), the total reservation territory being some 25,515 square miles (66,058 sq km).

The architects at DWL worked closely with user representatives to research and design the centre. It seems quite appropriate that the building which,

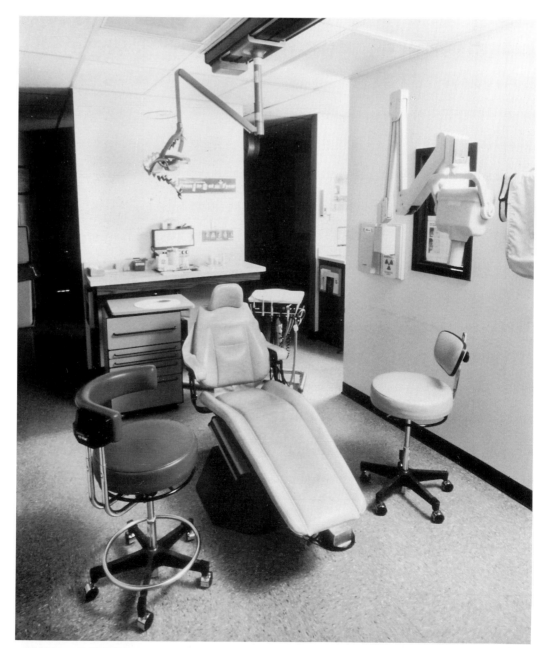

▷ Dental operatory.

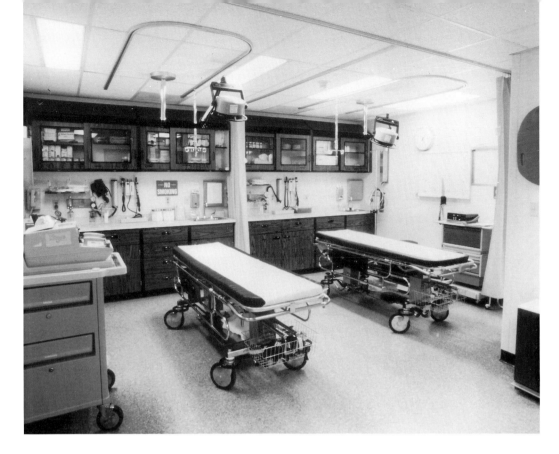

◁ *Treatment room in the emergency facility.*

after all, offers modern medical technology facilities including the dispensing of pharmaceutical drugs, should be a contemporary building. Anything else might have been viewed as patronizing. The concept of building as monument or institution is quite alien to the American-Indian spirit.

The building is a series of zones which relate to the different functional activities. Because of its remote location the centre includes an accident and emergency department. This has its own entrance which is placed discreetly at the rear of the building so that patients arriving for non-emergency care and treatment are not exposed to the arrival of ambulances and emergency cases.

As with the Straub Family Health Center, the entrance canopy serves as a useful transitional space between public and the semi-public area of the waiting room. The range of health services, from emergency treatment to health education, offer the opportunity for the patient population to have an integrated package of services.

Inscription House is an example of how primary health care can provide the vital dialogue with a community and deliver health services. Because of the care taken to involve and listen to the needs of its users, the centre is viewed as a valid resource. Its use depends upon the community accepting and utilizing the facilities. While there is a clash of building culture, this is still 'appropriate technology', as the building envelope can be maintained locally.

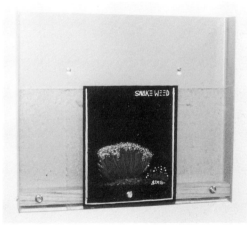

◁ *One of the symbols used for signage. This is the symbol for an examination room, one of several used in preference to room numbers.*

In other situation, such as Third World communities where the industrialized countries have planted modern technology in the form of hi-tech hospitals, they have in some cases failed because the indigenous population did not have the infrastructure to maintain and manage the facility.

Primary health care is at best 'care in the community by the community'. It is recognized that the historical/political circumstances of a reservation such as this are far from ideal, yet the architects who had to work within this existing situation have managed to provide a community facility without pretension and which respects the integrity of the functional requirements of the building as well as its patient population.

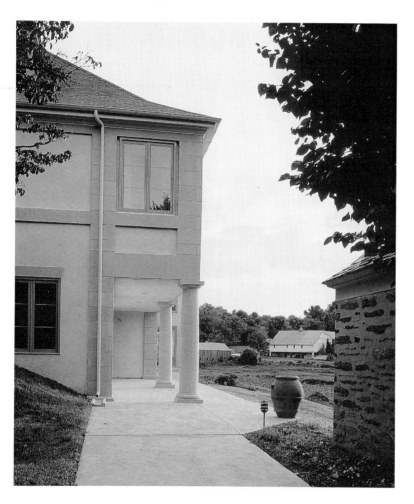

△ The Renfrew Center.
View to colonnade
entrance.

The Renfrew Center

Location:	**Philadelphia, Pennsylvania**
Completed:	**1985**
Type of facility:	**A new 42-bed care facility to treat eating disorders. Renovation of an existing 1920s residence into offices and treatment room**
Architects:	**Tony Atkin & Associates**
Client:	**Premier Medical Systems, Philadelphia, PA**
Gross floor area:	**1300 sq m (14,000 sq ft) new build. 650 sq m (7000 sq ft) renovated building**
Photography:	**Tom Bernard**

While our increasing knowledge and understanding of health care has eradicated certain forms of disease, new forms of health dysfunction have come into focus. Conditions such as AIDS and anorexia nervosa/bulimia, largely unheard of before, now present the challenge of new forms of treatment and care.

The nature of such conditions also require the creation of appropriate health environments, preferably within the community rather than a hospital setting. In recognition of this, two of the case studies within this book are drawn deliberately from the outer fringes of the definition of primary health care. The Renfrew Center in Philadelphia, USA, for the treatment of anorexia and bulimia, and the Masku Centre in Finland for the treatment and care of multiple sclerosis.

If the approach to primary health care as developed by the World Health Organization is to promote community participation, health promotion and joint work across different sectors, then the inclusion of these two case studies has direct relevance.

Architect's statement:

The Renfrew Center is the first private facility specifically dedicated to the treatment of the psychological eating disorders of anorexia nervosa and bulimia. Typically, these are treated in either hospital or psychiatric facilities, neither of which is equipped to treat both the behavioural and emotional routes to the problem. By treating only eating disorders, the owners sought to provide a higher more specific level of care at a lower cost. Tony Atkin & Associates were asked to design a facility which would adhere to the strict institutional requirements placed on health care centres, meet the programmatic need of the treatment method and yet create a building within a comfortable, residential atmosphere.

The site is in 27 acres of rolling countryside and contains an existing 1928 French-style manor house. The manor house has been modified for use as administrative and therapeutic offices. This existing building set the tone for the design of the new facility as well as the landscaping of the grounds. The original entrance to the site – a long avenue of trees – has been maintained as the access point for visitors and as a drop-off point. The new building and its gardens are reached by a paved path from the drop-off point. Staff parking is located behind the new building.

The treatment programme created for the Renfrew Center relies on individual contacts in which the patients establish goals for their treatment. Individual psychotherapy sessions are balanced by group interaction in art and physical therapy, communal meals and family counselling. The average length of treatment at the centre is between 45 and 60 days.

With this programme in mind, the clients envisaged a comfortable home-like environment. The 40–bed dormitory building houses living and recreational areas, kitchen and dining facilities, nursing control stations and patient suites. Renovation has eliminated the second-floor nursing staff and recreational rooms, and added several individual therapy rooms. Social interaction among the patients is encouraged by the placement of large, relaxing areas in the centre of each floor. These areas are open to their respective corridors and connected by an open stair.

The clients requested that the dining room be conveniently located, yet discreet, and not in constant view. The double-height room is situated at one end of the building, its entrance hidden by a change of direction in the corridor. A porch abuts the dining room and leads to the flower and vegetable gardens which are used as part of therapy.

The new building is constructed with exterior masonry bearing walls, structural steel framing, steel joists, deck floors and wood roof trusses. Exterior finishes include stucco, car stones, steel columns, wood trims, wood windows and composition shingle. Interior partitions are fire resistant, dry wall and metal studs. Interior finishes

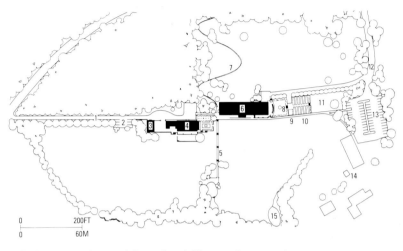

1. Existing entrance road	6. New residence building	11. Outdoor recreation
2. Visitor parking	7. Hiking path	12. Service road
3. Allied therapy	8. Flower garden	13. Staff parking
4. Administration and therapy	9. Garden shed	14. Existing barn and farm buildings
5. New path to pool	10. Vegetable garden	15. Retention pond

include simple wood cornice mouldings and other woodwork, carpet and wood flooring.

△ Location plan. The site at Renfrew Farm, originally the estate of Mrs Samuel F. Houston, was designed by Robert McGoodwin in 1929. The existing manor house is used with minor modifications for administrative and therapeutic offices.

Main activity areas

Patient care & community spaces

Allied therapy rooms
Living rooms (× 2)
Dining room
Small dining room
Reception room
Terrace
Double bedrooms (× 19)
Single bedrooms (× 6) previously designated 'time out' rooms

Staff

Administration (in existing manor house)
Nursing stations (× 2)
Kitchen
Service entrance
Staff offices (in existing manor house)

69

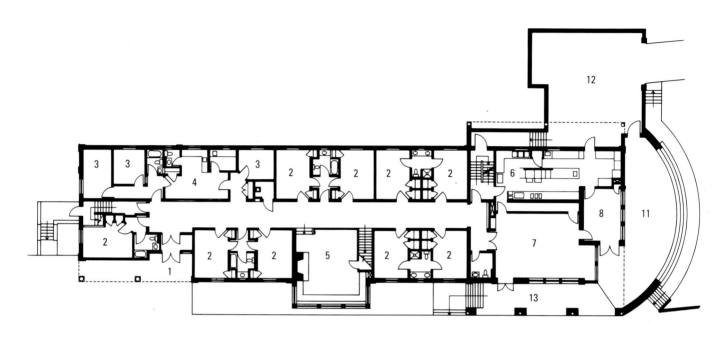

0 _____ 30FT
0 _____ 10M

Ground floor plan
1 Entrance
2 Double bedroom
3 Time out room in use as single bedrooms
4 Nurses' station in use as art room/coffee corner
5 Living room
6 Kitchen
7 Dining room

8 Adjunct dining room
9 Recreation room
10 Open below
11 Terrace
12 Service yard
13 Veranda

△ Ground-floor plan.

▽ First-floor plan.

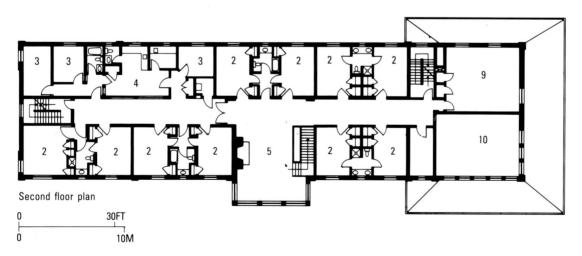

Second floor plan

0 _____ 30FT
0 _____ 10M

THE LIBRARY
GUILDFORD COLLEGE
of Further and Higher Education

Comment

The Renfrew Center stands on the threshold of a completely new type of care facility. It is the first of its kind, departing from the institutional norm, both in operational and architectural design.

Anorexia nervosa and bulimia have only recently emerged as a major health problem. Forms of treatment tend to take account of behavioural, physical and – most importantly – the psychological aspects of a patient's makeup. As with AIDS there is growing concern that there are few (if any) appropriate facilities which are designed and managed to offer an appropriate and supportive environment for treatment.

Such conditions cannot effectively be treated within the medical/clinical environment of a hospital. They warrant a more community-based setting, removed from the stigma of an institution.

The site in Upper Roxborugh, Pennsylvania, is isolated yet not remote. The architects undertook only minor alterations to the original manor house, retaining the main rooms for administrative or therapy use. The site offered only a limited option. The manor house is informally situation, set not at the crown but into the side of a steep hill. The drive slips by the front facade and the carriage house court, manor house and terrace are strung out in one long line along the road. The entrance to the new wing, hidden behind the drive's original end wall, is still more informal and less imposing. The new building set back further into the hillside defers to the main house, echoing its roof silhouettes and detail. In matching the manor house the architects not only complement the original, but disguise their own structure complying with the client's request that Renfrew appear residential.

For all its reassuring domestic detail, Renfrew is a licensed rehabilitation centre as is evident from the interior, more so than the exterior. In the absence of a specific role model the architects relied on state standards developed for substance-abuse (drug and alcohol treatment) centres. They also followed the treatment schedule devised for Renfrew by Dr Steven Emmett of Boston quite

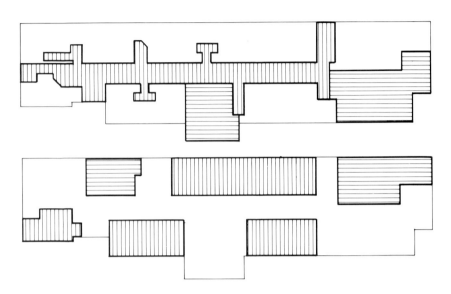

closely. Emmett's programme is based upon individual therapeutic 'contracts'. Patients set their own goals for treatment with staff guidance, group interaction, physical and art therapy, communal meals and family counselling – all group activities – in addition to individual psychotherapy sessions, carried out over a 45 to 60 day stay. Thus the Renfrew 'dorm' has as its heart a pair of large living rooms that are the focus for social interaction and group therapy sessions. The main stair, a natural

△ *Main circulation routes, ground floor.*

△ *Main functional areas, ground floor.*

▽ *Main circulation routes, first floor.*

▽ *Main functional areas, first floor.*

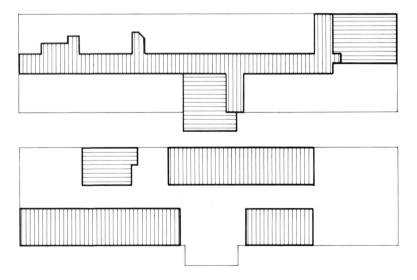

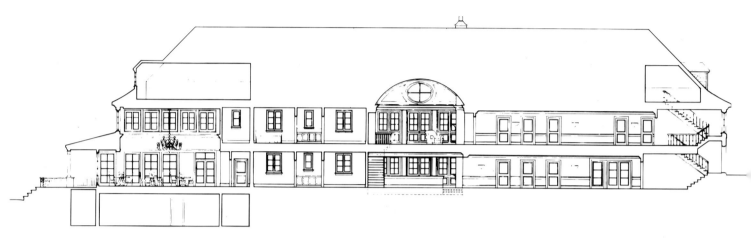

△ *Section through length of facility.*

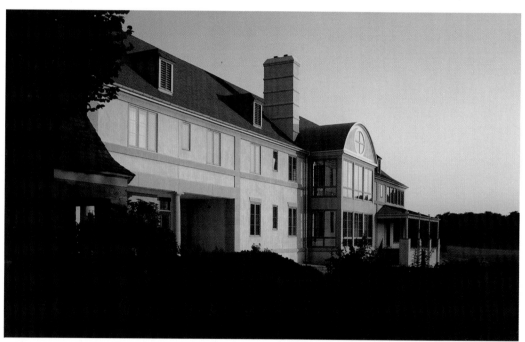

▷ *West elevation at sunset.*

▷ *View of new facility with original manor house in background.*

means of social contact, opens directly into these rooms. The units themselves all doubles with shared baths are deliberately furnished and finished in a non-institutional fashion. The only hospital item is a call-button. Bedrooms open on to the corridor whose wide proportions (in compliance with wheelchair regulations) afford additional opportunities for casual contact. These corridors in turn open directly into the living rooms, a critical connection, and one that required amendment to the standard code.

The 'time out' rooms, designed for monitored isolation, function as special units for patients who require the privacy of a single room. Renfrew's clinical director, Dr Leonard S. Levitz, finds the glass-enclosed nursing stations (carried over from the substance-abuse code) too hospital-like. Neither station is used as designed, serving instead

72

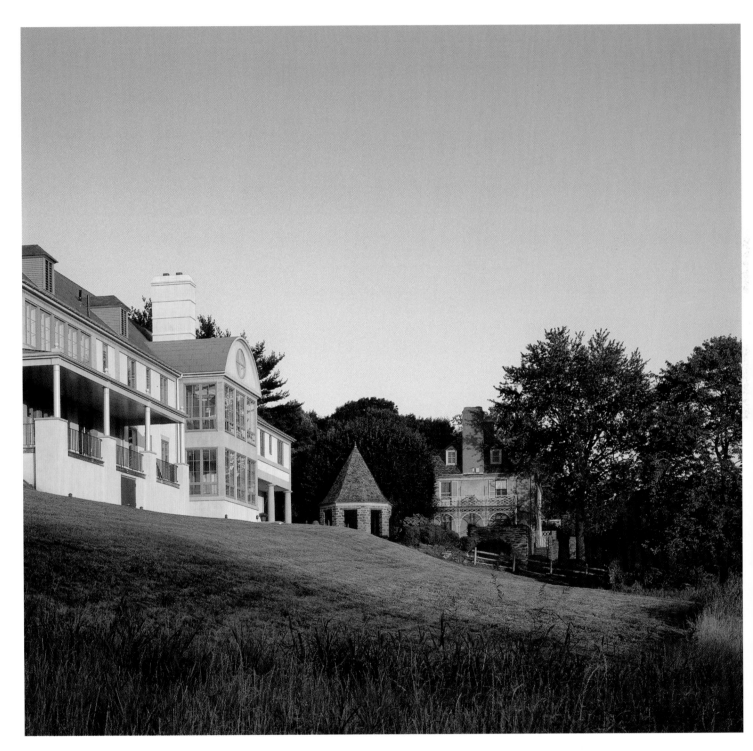

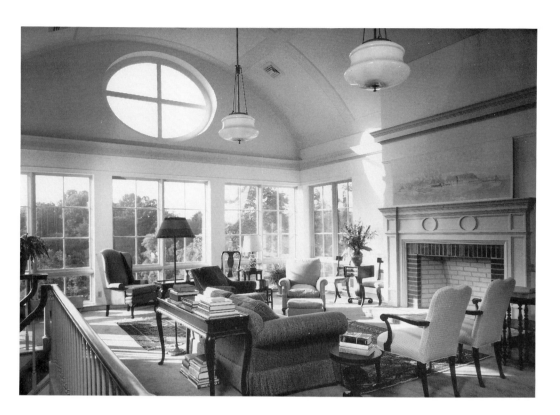

▷ *The upstairs living room.*

as impromptu art or coffee corner, fully accessible to patients.

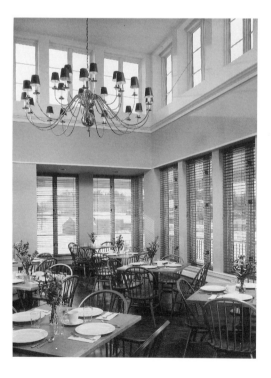

▷ *The main dining room.*

While it is too early to assess the success of Renfrew's programme, the current population of 18 (60 total since it opened) is ahead of schedule. In November 1985 the client bought 19 additional acres adjacent to the farm, and they are now exploring a number of possible programmes including a conference centre for the study of eating disorders or a stress management clinic.

As the first of its type, the fact that certain rooms are being utilized for purposes other than those intended in the programme is to be expected. The importance for any such buildings is to have the ability (as at Renfrew) to flex and change to adapt to evolving work patterns.

While Renfrew has, as yet, no imitators, the centre has generated considerable national interest and enquiries from as far afield as Australia, Italy and Israel, suggesting that this type of small-scale specialized care offered potentially on a community/regional basis may be the way of the future.

Note
The above comments are based on an article by Darallce D. Boles previously published in *Progressive Architecture* **LXVII** (4), April 1986.

Japan

Population 1990:	**123.87 million**
Percentage of population aged 65 plus:	**11.4**
Population estimated 2020:	**132.61 million**
Percentage of population aged 65 plus (2020):	**20.8**
Health care expenditure in pounds per person:	**625**
Health care expressed as percentage of GNP:	**5.2**

(Source: Compendium of Health Statistics, Office of Health Economics, London, UK.)

Japan's standard of living and the state of its nation's health have improved dramatically over the past 40 years. In 1989 Japan recorded the world's lowest infant mortality rate and highest longevity figures.

Yet the structure of the health service system is complex, involving compulsory health insurance via several health insurance plans. These are either paid for by the individual or employers will often make contributions to cover the employee but not necessarily his or her family. Medical services tend to be based upon a fee for service with nationally set charges whilst health education programmes are free of charge. The concept of a primary health care centre has been part of Japan's health care culture since the 1930s.

In common with other industrialized countries the network of hospitals and attention to acute care has developed the most rapidly and has absorbed most of Japan's health care expenditure.

Other factors have also influenced the type of health services now required in Japan. These include:

- An increasingly ageing population bringing with it the need to provide long-term health care for chronic disorders.
- A shift in emphasis away from the traditional treatment of communicable diseases (cholera, dysentery) towards preventive medicine and health education programmes.
- A greater emphasis on pre- and post-natal care.

Part of this change in emphasis has been reflected in the increasing development of primary health care, a network of health centres providing the core of this programme.

Japan's health service has traditionally needed to respond mainly to control and treatment of communicable diseases. However, the industrialization of the country combined with Western influence (including diet) has brought with it a high incidence of cerebrovascular disease, malignant neoplasms and heart disease.

At present the concepts of public health and community medicine education are still viewed as separate in terms of the facilities provided for each.

Public health education services including immunization, maternal care and child health guidance are largely available from health centres. Medical treatment is however only available via hospitals or clinics. Public health programmes were founded in 1870 to combat the often catastrophic cholera or dysentery epidemics. Prevention was emphasized by enforcing regulations on food, hygiene and environmental sanitation. As the rate of epidemics subsided and such diseases became more controlled, public health programmes became more involved in promoting maternal and child health and the prevention of tuberculosis. Such common conditions were seen as affecting the mass of the population and were therefore perceived within a framework of public health and the responsibility of the state.

In 1937 the Health Centre Law was enacted. The term 'health centres' in Japan, however, referred to a government health education guidance agency for the benefit of the nation's health. Health centres were not seen as a place for medical treatment. The Health Centre Law was revised in 1947, giving further encouragement to the creation of more health centres. Under the 1947 legislation, local government areas including the major cities were required to establish health centres.

Today there are over 900 health centres in Japan funded by the state and offering free services, but only in the field of preventive medicine and health education.

Medical consultations and treatment will normally take place within a physician's clinic or at a hospital. Such services are not free and have to be paid for via medical insurance. Although medical care operates within the private sector, provisions and standards are regulated as part of the administrative functions of the state health centres.

There is, therefore, co-ordination between the state and the private sector to ensure a balance in the nation's health care system between demand, cost and quality of service.

A physician's clinic typically comprises a single family doctor working with a nurse (often his wife) within a facility which would also accommodate up to 19 beds. Often the doctor and his family will have residence on the site and will be on call 24 hours, thus offering a dedicated and very personal care service. It would function as a hybrid of a doctor's surgery and a small community hospital. The range of services range from general practice to obstetrical care and surgical procedures. The physician's clinic therefore plays a vital role within Japan's primary health care system.

Hospitals have recognized the demand for a more community-based primary care service and have begun to develop medical centres utilizing their corporate finance structures and effecting an economy of scale in building management, servicing and marketing.

This has led hospital-based clinics to enter and compete with the physician's clinics. Recognition that such conflict could be against the national interest has led to a policy that actually encourages hospitals to refer primary health care patients to local clinics (a reversal of the United Kingdom system of GPs referring to hospitals). To balance this, physician's clinics, which previously had no links with hospitals, are now encouraged to refer patients who would benefit from more intensive and specialized treatment to the hospital. In each case this policy is backed via the financial incentives of a flat referral fee paid by the state to either party.

The physician's clinic may not always have the benefit of state-of-the-art diagnosis and treatment technology. However, because the cost of care is often cheaper, the clinic system remains an attractive option for both patient and sponsor.

Japan's primary health care system has its tradition in the health centre as a national network for preventive medicine, guidance and health education. Primary medical treatment remains based upon the physician's clinic which may well become more allied and integrated with the technical and staff resources of the hospital.

References

Levin, P.J. (1989) Health care in the balance: Japanese eurythmy. *Hospitals & Health Services Administration*, **34**(3), 311–323.

Miura, K. (1988) The roles of health centres for the community health in Japan. *World Hospitals*, **24**(1), 39–47.

Hirayama Clinic

Location: **Tohgane (Chiba Prefecture)**
Completed: **1987**
Type of facility: **Physician's clinic with a ward of 19 beds and doctor's residence**
Architect: **Yasumitsu Matsunaga/SKM Architects & Planners Inc.**
Client: **Dr Osamu Hirayama (surgeon)**
Gross floor area: **900.94 sq m (9700 sq ft)**
Photography: **Ryusi Miyamoto**

Architect's statement:
Yasumitsu Matsunaga

The physician's clinic had been established for 40 years. When we started the design for the new clinic in 1985 my main concern was initially nothing other than a functional response to the client's programme and the site's analysis: a surgery clinic with 19 beds and a doctor's residence attached to it looking upon an existing pond with maximum capacity for parking in the front yard.

However, while teaching at Washington University in St Louis in the United States as a design critic in 1986 a new view of architecture arose in my mind, looking into the value of catastrophe, chaos and intuition; this in contrast to that of harmony, reason and order established in the age of classicism in Europe as was studied by Michael Foucault.[1] Thus the initial design of the clinic was transformed little by little. First of all I became aware of the mental effects of physical space upon mental care. Recent studies have revealed that good medical care depends unexpectedly highly upon the mental state of the patient. Intuitively I felt a desire to wrap a tender and soothing space over the site with a tuft of flying wings. The exterior was enclosed in metallic panels which by contrast enhanced the softness of the

▽ *Hirayama Clinic, Tohgane, Japan.*

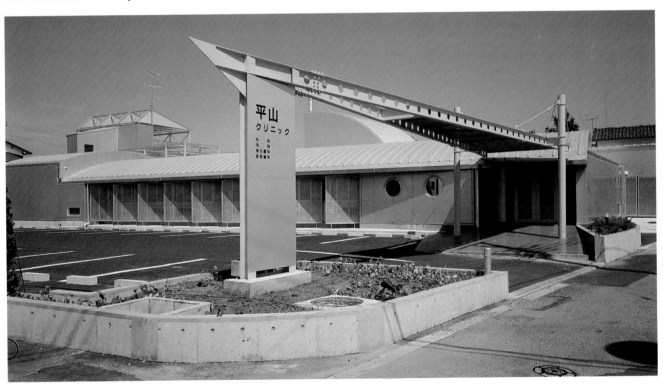

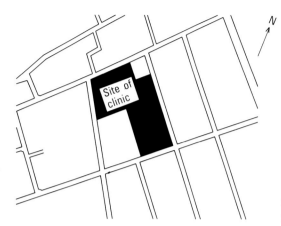

▷ *Location plan.*

▽ *Ground-floor plan. The doctor's residence is two-storey with the second bedroom on the upper floor.*

interior as well as symbolizing the precision of the doctor's expertise. In the patients' rooms (where they spend most of their time) we provided deep eaves, a wide window, loft ceiling and indirect lighting without optical disturbance to allow for better rest.

Four triangular yellow flags on the roof of the residential section convey the image of sails flying in the wind from the nearby Pacific Ocean, and

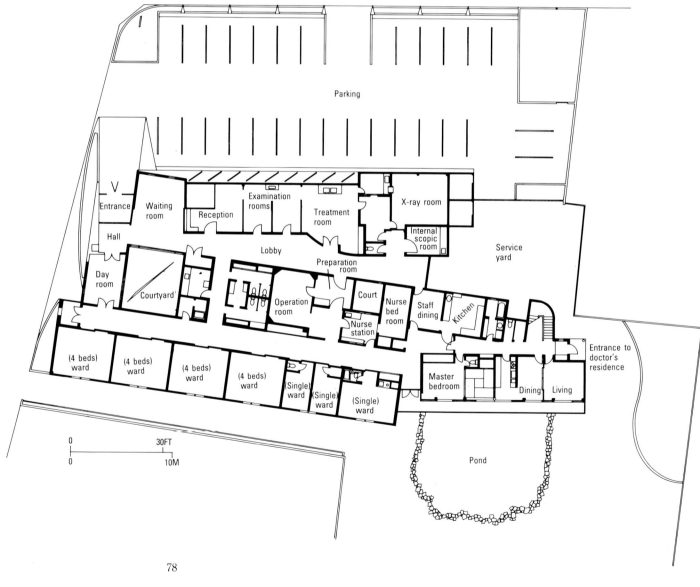

correspond to the triangular canopy at the entrance.

Nothing could have flattered us more than the news from the doctor that patients would be reluctant to leave his clinic even after their illness was cured.

Comment

A 'prefecture' is one of 47 administrative areas within Japan similar in terms to a health district. Tohgane is located in the Chiba prefecture, approximately 31 miles (50 km) to the east of Tokyo.

It is a rapidly growing area located on the Pacific Ocean. The site lies within a mixed-use area near the Tohgane railway station and the existing guest house and pond.

From entering the site the dramatic yellow canopy clearly marks the point of entry. It not only offers the visual key to locating the entrance but also provides shelter to patients transferring from vehicles. The entrance canopy structure is also effectively utilized to display the name of the clinic. From the entry lobby the reception desk is located past the waiting area. A screen allows supervision of the waiting area from reception.

The plan clearly follows the three functions of the clinic:

- Consultation – examination – treatment
- Surgical procedures
- In-patient accommodation

The consultation – examination – treatment sector fronts on to the car park and includes an X-ray facility. The surgical section of the clinic forms the spine of the building containing the operating room, preparation rooms and staff rooms including an overnight stay area for the nurse on duty. The patient care area forms the main wing with a combination of four-bed and single-bed units plus a day room.

Finally, the doctor's two bedroom residence; this has a separate entrance but is linked to the clinic on

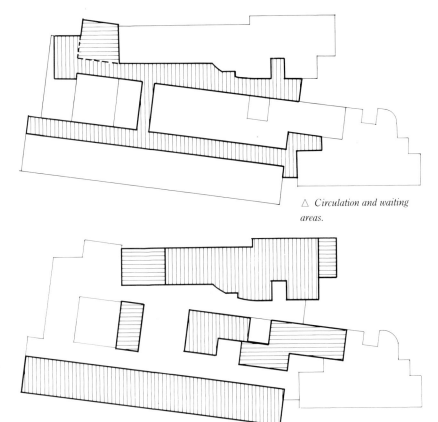

△ *Circulation and waiting areas.*

△ *Staff and patient care areas.*

the patient bed wing. With the exception of the second bedroom, all accommodation is on the ground floor.

The work of the clinic will tend to be a combination of out-patients/consultation and in-patients/post-operative care.

From reception patients will wait to see the physician or nurse, and will then be shown to one of the examination rooms for initial consultation. If necessary, samples and X-rays will be taken. For out-patient sessions the patient would then leave the clinic without having to penetrate the building any further.

For surgical procedures involving only day care, patients will be taken to the preparation room and then to the operation room. After the operation patients would recover in one of the bedrooms and in the case of minor operations could leave the same day. Because the physician lives on site the quality and attention of service will be high. There

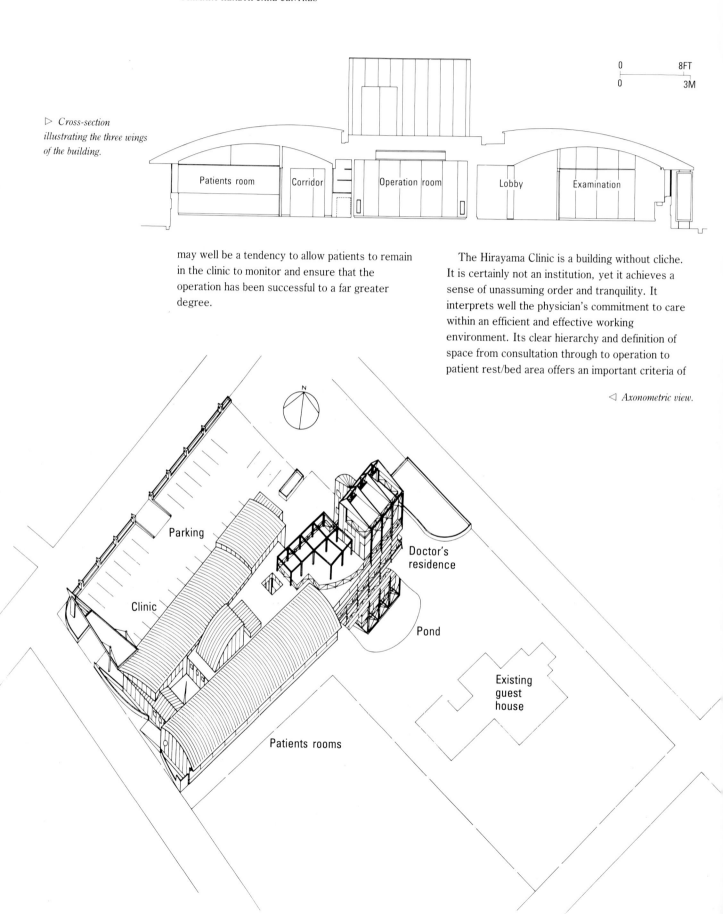

0   8FT
0   3M

▷ *Cross-section*
illustrating the three wings
of the building.

Patients room   Corridor   Operation room   Lobby   Examination

may well be a tendency to allow patients to remain
in the clinic to monitor and ensure that the
operation has been successful to a far greater
degree.

The Hirayama Clinic is a building without cliche.
It is certainly not an institution, yet it achieves a
sense of unassuming order and tranquility. It
interprets well the physician's commitment to care
within an efficient and effective working
environment. Its clear hierarchy and definition of
space from consultation through to operation to
patient rest/bed area offers an important criteria of

◁ *Axonometric view.*

N

Parking

Doctor's
residence

Clinic

Pond

Existing
guest
house

Patients rooms

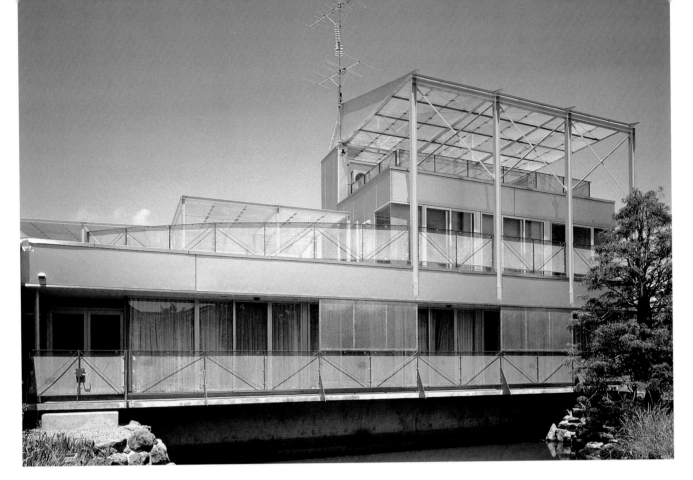

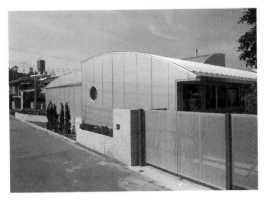

◁ *View from south-west looking on to patients' room (to the right).*

△ *View towards doctor's residence.*

▽ *Aerial view showing the clinic in the context of its site.*

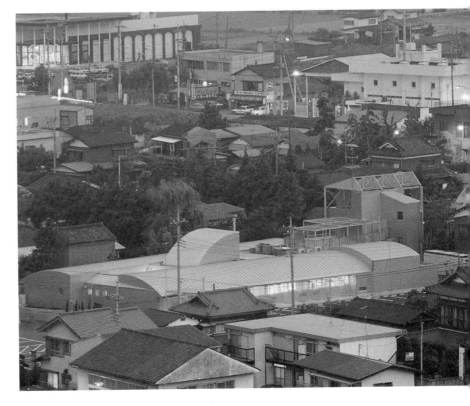

special order, important within this system of health care and treatment. The internal finishes can be perceived as rather hard, especially the floor. Perhaps a carpet, at least in the circulation areas, could have alleviated this impression.

Nevertheless, in the context of its culture and the framework of the site it is an entirely appropriate building which is well liked by both staff and patients. As a primary health care building it is able to bridge the gap between physician and hospital. As such it follows the function of the GP hospital favoured by some United Kingdom practices; the inclusion of in-patient beds is, after all, a reflection of the Dawson Report for Health Centres of the 1920s.

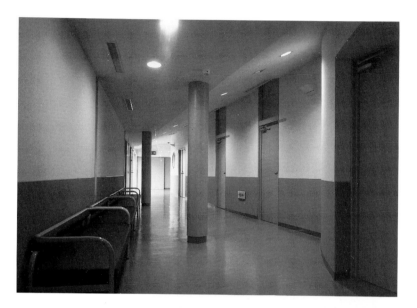

△ *Circulation area with treatment suite to the right looking back towards the entrance.*

▷ *Courtyard as viewed from waiting room.*

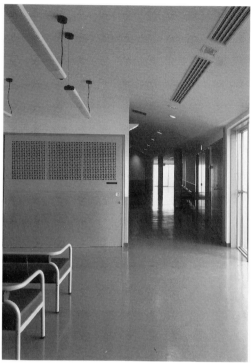

△ *Waiting room with courtyard to the right.*

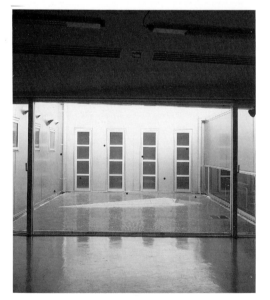

Main activity areas (excluding doctor's residence)

Patients
Waiting room
Day room
WC

Patient care
Examination rooms (× 2)
Treatment room
Operating room
Preparation room
Patients' room 4 beds (× 4)
Patients' room single (× 3)
Internal scopic room
Nurse station
Nurse bedroom
Staff dining
Kitchen

Reference

1. *Japan Architect*, No. 357, January, p. 5.

The United Kingdom

Population 1990: **56.19 million**
Percentage of population aged 65 plus: **15.6**
Population estimated year 2020: **56.08 million**
Percentage of population aged 65 plus (2020): **17.8**
Health care expenditure in pounds per person: **423**
Health care expenditure expressed as percentage of GNP: **5.8**

(Source: Compendium of Health Statistics, Office of Health Economics, London, UK.)

Primary health care in the UK is delivered from a variety of premises ranging from converted shop units, doctors' own homes, to modern purpose-built primary care facilities. It is only recently that primary health care services have come to occupy a more prominent position in the general field of debate in health policy.

Primary care has traditionally been a service which has suffered from a lack of co-ordination, due to the various paymasters of primary health care practitioners. For example, independent contractors, which include general practitioners, dentists and opticians to salaried community health staff which include district nurses and health visitors, to salaried local authority staff which includes social workers.

Since the 1980s there has been a greater emphasis on primary health care, but this has been linked with consumerism, accountability and value for money. Furthermore, in an attempt to improve co-ordination between the various bodies involved in primary health care major organizational shifts have taken place in both planning and management.

In 1985, Family Practitioner Committees (FPC) now known as Family Health Services Authorities (FHSA) (the body which administers the services of general practitioners, dentists and opticians) became independent authorities whose remit included additional management and planning responsibilities. Some FPCs undertook surveys of existing practice premises, particularly in the inner

cities, to gauge overall existing standards and to encourage, where possible, improvements. As a result, many FHSAs are well advanced in identifying their contractors' services and facilities in order to forward plan to a strategic level, in collaboration with other health authorities, particularly with regards to immunization, vaccination and child health surveillance.

However, because this is a new approach such collaboration will need to develop, as can be seen in the first building study. A lack of collaboration can lead to missed opportunities and potentially wasted resources. A further debate concerning primary health care services and its problem of narrow definition is set out in the 1987 White Paper. Demographic changes and early discharge from hospitals and day care arrangements will increase the current trend towards general practitioners and their health staff providing continuing care in the community for patients with chronic disorders. In the United States and Scandinavia this is beginning to lead to community-based facilities specifically serving such patients, but functioning as a resource centre for primary health care. (See Renfrew Center, Philadelphia, page 68 and Masku Centre, Finland, page 139.)

The new organizational changes must respond to the changing demands on primary care. In the United Kingdom more and more hospitals have undertaken day surgery and reduced the length of stay in acute wards since the 1970s. In addition the Government is promoting a greater emphasis on provision of care in the community rather than in centralized institutions for patients with long-term disabilities. This also applies to the increasing number of older people requiring long-term support, to be undertaken in the community, rather than in institutions.

This, combined with the general view that primary health care facilities are the most appropriate vehicle for preventive health programmes, has brought the services and facilities of primary health care practitioners into sharp focus. In 1987 the Government published a White Paper for implementing the restructuring of primary health care services. In 1990 a new Contract of Service for General Practitioners was put into operation.[1]

The key objectives of the White Paper and the 1990 Contract are:

- To make services more responsible to the consumer
- To raise standards of care
- To promote health and prevent illness
- To give patients the widest range of choice in obtaining high quality primary care services
- To improve value for money
- To enable clarification of priorities for Family Practitioner Services in relation to the rest of the nation's health service.[2]

Each of these implies better standards of building facilities. In particular, the Family Health Services Authorities are being encouraged to play a more active role in administrative and planning of such services and facilities, including:

- Setting of targets for preventive services
- Inspecting and monitoring standards of premises
- Provision of more comprehensive information on practitioner services
- The eliciting of public comments on the quality of those services as provided.

In 1991 GP fund-holding was introduced whereby practices with at least 11,000 patients were offered the opportunity to be given a fixed budget of primary and secondary care in order to:

- Improve the quality of GP services
- Help GPs develop their practices for patients' benefits
- Give GPs greater control over use of resources
- Encourage hospitals to be more responsive to the needs of GPs and their patients

The minimum requirement has since dropped to 9,000 patients, with further programmes expected to allow practices of 4,500 patients to become eligible as fund holders.[3]

The intended benefits of funding holding are: reduced hospital waiting times, greater communication/cooperation between consultant and GP and reduced costs.

Because of the independent contractual status of the GP, the method by which primary care centres are designed and funded has followed two distinct paths:

1 Buildings directly funded, built and owned by Area Health Authorities. These have often been referred to as 'health centres'. As stated in Chapter 2, the provision of such facilities was embodied in the National Health Service Act of 1946. As buildings owned and managed by Area Health Authorities, GPs as independent contractors have to pay to the Authority rent for the space they use. They are thus tenants, not owners, of the building.

2 Buildings directly funded, built and owned or leased by GPs. As a result of financial assistance programmes administered by FHSAs (formerly FPCs) known as 'improvement grant' or 'cost rent reimbursement',[4] an increasing number of GPs have elected to develop their own practice premises. The GP therefore may well be the owner and manager of such a facility. Where doctors combine to form group practices, then suitable accommodation can facilitate the concept of the primary health care team. However, the cost and availability of land – combined with the cash limiting of both cost rent and improvement grant programmes – is severely restricting the opportunities for primary health care, particularly in the inner cities, which is often the area of critical need (see page 178).

As the focus moves towards both primary and community care, as recommended by the Tomlinson Report for London (1992), so it will be essential that adequate funding can support and encourage adequate and appropriate premises for its effective delivery.

References

1. Marks, L. (1988) *Promoting Better Health? An Analysis of the Government's Programme for Primary Health Care*, King's Fund Institute, London.

2. CM249 (1987) *Promoting Better Health: The Government's Programme for Improving Primary Health Care*, HMSO, London.

3. Pirie, A. and Kelly, M. (1992) 'Fund-holding: A practice guide', Radcliffe Medical Press, Oxford.

4. For further information on cost rent and improvement grant programmes see Health Building Note 46. (1991) 'General medical practice premises for the provision of primary care services': NHS Estates. HMSO, London. Chisholm J. (Ed.) 'Making Sense of the Cost Rent Scheme' (1992) Radcliffe Medical Press, Oxford.

The John Telford Clinic

Location: **Ilford, Essex**
Completed: **1989**
Type of facility: **Health authority clinic**
Architects: **Avanti Architects Ltd**
Client: **North East Thames Regional Health Authority (project team including representatives from regional and district health authorities)**
Gross floor area: **792 sq m (8522 sq ft)**
Photography: **Martin Charles**

Architect's statement:
John Allan, Avanti Architects Ltd

The brief called for clinical facilities for health education and child health programmes, a dental surgery, speech therapy and chiropody clinic. There was a need for office accommodation for administrative staff, health visitors and district nurses and other para-medicals. In addition were the requisite reception, waiting and support services, and car parking areas for the above.

The client user group indicated a need for flexibility of operation. For example health education and child health accommodation were to be operated in evening sessions when the offices and other clinics were closed. It would also be desirable to be able to close off the latter two groups of rooms independently. Such criteria, together with the nature of the site (a cul-de-sac approached from the south), implied a single level ground-floor cruciform plan. Two wings are provided for the two groups with clinical requirements, and the third for staff. A short entrance wing contains the pram park and entrance to central reception and waiting areas. This arrangement produces four external spaces which are developed respectively as:

- Entrance approach/privacy strip
- A staff car park (screened by the entrance and overlooked by the staff offices)

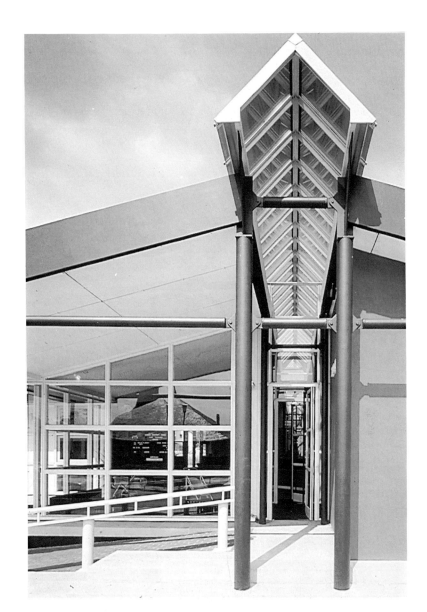

- Gardens for clinic
- Gardens for staff

△ *The John Telford Clinic, Ilford, Essex.*

Immediately to the south of the clinic is a general practice surgery which was built shortly before this scheme was initiated. A co-ordination of services is intended to provide a comprehensive primary health care facility.

85

▷ The John Telford Clinic is located within a comparatively run down area of Ilford, a suburb to the north-east of London. It is well positioned in relation to local housing, transport and other communal facilities.

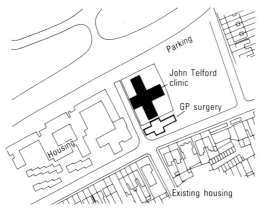

Parking

John Telford clinic

GP surgery

Housing

Existing housing

Design approach

Although the clinic is located close to the new Ilford town centre, the main catchment area to the south is uniformly suburban. The architectural character of the scheme seeks to reconcile the public status of the building with the domestic scale of its surroundings. The height and profile are therefore consistent with its neighbours, while the expression and materials are differentiated.

The plan form aims to provide good legibility and supervision while the section is designed to maximize distribution of natural light and

▷ The plan is based upon a simple yet sophisticated cruciform arrangement. The reception area forms the central pivot to the plan, so it is possible to visually supervise both entrance and main patient circulation routes.

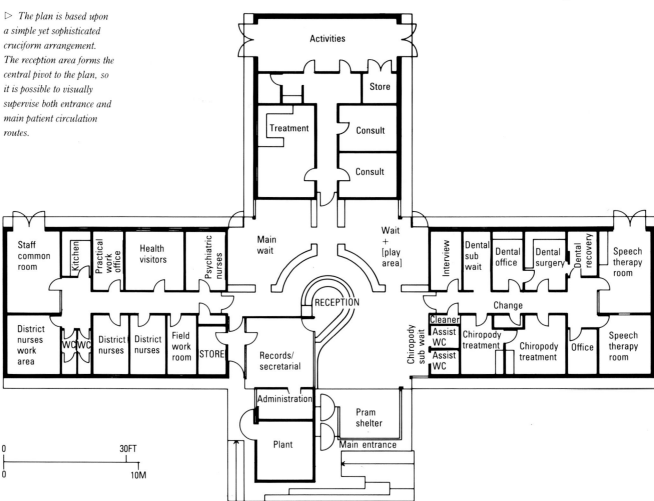

Activities

Store

Treatment

Consult

Consult

Staff common room · Kitchen · Practical work office · Health visitors · Psychiatric nurses · Main wait · Wait + [play area] · Interview · Dental sub wait · Dental office · Dental surgery · Dental recovery · Speech therapy room

RECEPTION

Change

District nurses work area · WC · WC · District nurses · District nurses · Field work room · STORE · Records/ secretarial · Chiropody sub wait · Cleaner · Assist WC · Assist WC · Chiropody treatment · Chiropody treatment · Office · Speech therapy room

Administration

Pram shelter

Plant

Main entrance

0 ———— 30FT
0 ———— 10M

THE LIBRARY
GUILDFORD COLLEGE
of Further and Higher Education

ventilation. All waiting areas have external views and all main rooms are day-lit from two sides, the interior by means of a clerestory transmitting borrowed light from the central spine roof light. Patients/visitors are directed to the appropriate clinic at reception. A separate staff entrance beside the entrance wing enables staff to enter and leave the building independently. The reception area is designed to allow for sales of welfare foods/ enquiries, etc. Visitors using these services need not penetrate far into the building. Records are kept centrally in the reception office. The plant room is placed in the north facing half of the entrance wing, with easy service access from the road/car park.

Methods of construction

The building consists of a steel frame superstructure on a reinforced concrete raft slab. The external walls employ a purpose design standardized timber screen with window/panel infill and blockwork back-up wall, which is detailed internally as a parameter service duct. The roof is covered with a proprietory profiled aluminium interlocking sheet system used in conjunction with a purpose design aluminium rain-water disposal system draining to the three bank gables. The roof light is of double-glazed toughened/laminated solar control glass. There are no roof penetrations whatsoever. The internal partitions are of non-load-bearing blockwork to eaves level with timber stud work above. External windows and doors are aluminium colour coated.

All furniture and furnishings were chosen to be consistent with the architectural design of the building.

Main activity areas

Patients
Entrance lobby
Pram/cycle shelter
Waiting area (× 2)

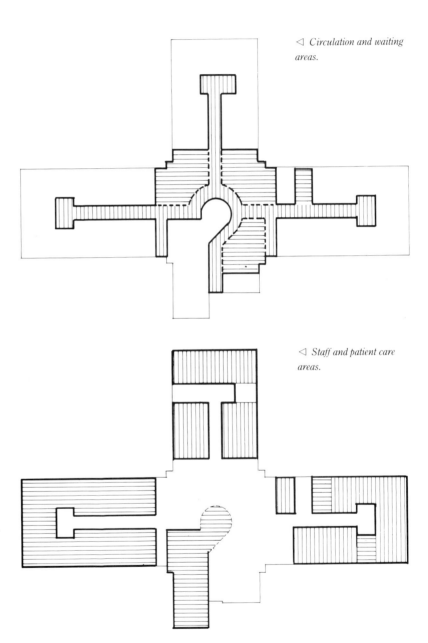

◁ Circulation and waiting areas.

◁ Staff and patient care areas.

Play area
Dental sub-wait
Chiropody change
Chiropody sub-wait
Assisted WCs (× 2)
Specimen WC

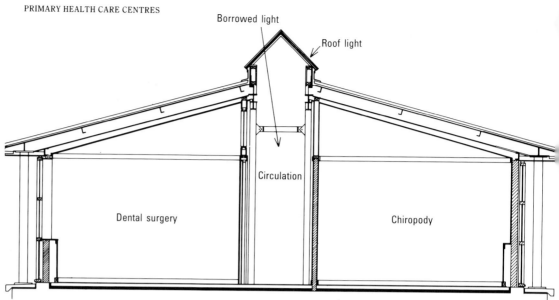

Borrowed light

Roof light

Circulation

Dental surgery

Chiropody

▷ *As a single-storey building the architects fully exploited the opportunity of introducing top lighting above the circulation areas. This further emphasized and gave clarity to the activity of movement around the building.*

▷ *Main entrance facade. The patients' entrance is inviting and a refreshing contrast to the immediate environment.*

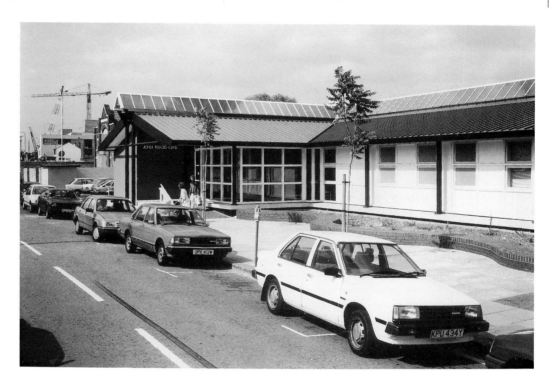

Patient care areas
Consulting rooms (× 2)
Dental surgery
Dental recovery
Chiropody treatment (× 2)
Speech therapy treatment
Speech therapy play
Interview
Health education area
Treatment area

Staff areas
Reception
Records admin
Admin office
Dental office
Speech therapy office
District nurses (× 2)
District nurse practical work teacher
Health visitors
Health visitors/fieldwork teacher

Community psychiatric nurse
Stores (× 2)
Staff lounge
Staff kitchen
Cleaner's store
Staff WCs
Staff entrance
Plant room

Comment

The John Telford Clinic is located within a comparatively run down area of Ilford, a suburb to the north-east of London. It is well positioned in relation to local housing and its accessibility to other local transport and community facilities.

Its location therefore sets it very much within the local fabric as a community resource. The adjacent GP Unit by sheer proximity should at least encourage co-operation among the primary health care team. Ideally both buildings should have been planned simultaneously at least to allow a physical link between the two facilities.

The entrance to the building is expressed through bold use of colour and a clarity of architectural form. It provides an inviting and

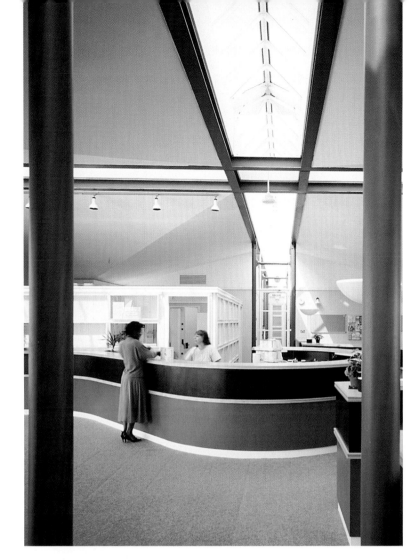

△ *The main reception area.*

◁ *The activities of the reception area at the clinic also include the sale and distribution of baby foods and supplies.*

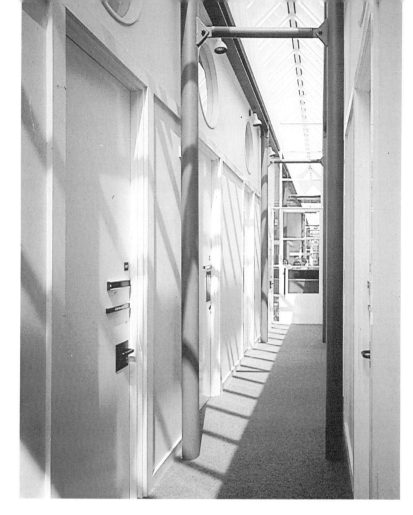

◁ *Typical corridor detail.*
The Reception area remains
visible from the corridor
thus offering the all

important clues to assist a
patient's orientation within
the building.

refreshing contrast from the otherwise nondescript surroundings. The building therefore does not attempt (or want) to blend in with the local environment. Instead its simple yet innovative form almost echoes the design philosophy of the Finsbury Health Centre (page 4). It is interesting to note that the architects have an intimate knowledge of the Finsbury Health Centre, as they are due to be involved in its planned restoration.

From the street the building is accessed either via a gently sloping ramp or a few steps. The entrance itself enjoys the protection of the main roof structure.

The pram shelter benefits from being contained within the building 'envelope'. It can be visually supervised from the reception of one of the waiting areas.

From the point of entry the reception desk is immediately identified. Its position ensures a pivotal control over both entrance circulation and waiting areas. Office administration, although adjacent to the reception, is located in a separate area. This safeguards any confidential files or records from unauthorised view.

There are three waiting areas, each accommodating two distinct types of patients:

- Main waiting area for consulting and treatment room
- Chiropody sub-wait
- Dental sub-wait

The simple plan and clarity of design contribute substantially to the uncomplicated circulation pattern. The reception desk, the first main feature identified upon entering the building, retains its focus as a route-finder. It is the crossroads of the four circulation routes. It can also be seen upon leaving a room, so orientation back to the waiting area/reception/exit is straightforward. The top lighting of the circulation routes reinforces this clarity.

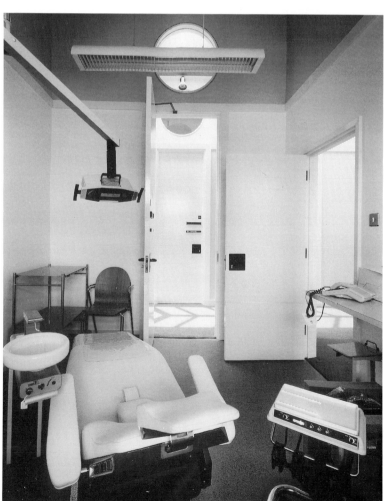

◁ *Dental suite. Note*
circular clerestory light
above the door. The
architects have provided

every opportunity for
natural light to filter
through and within the
building.

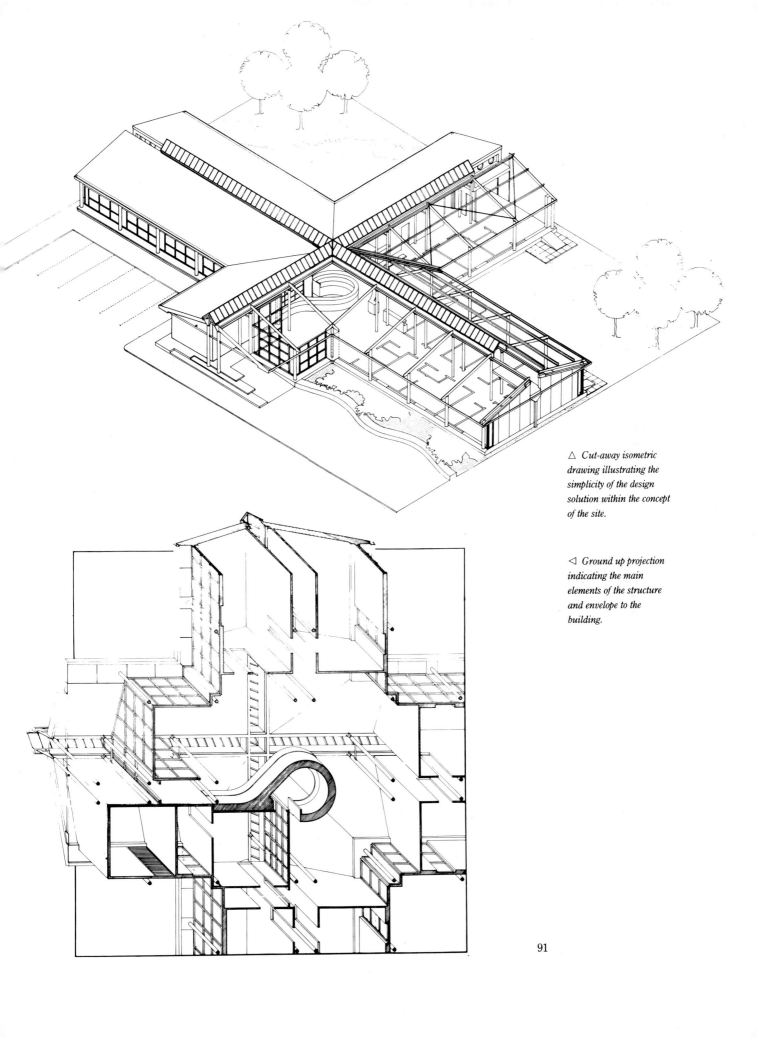

△ Cut-away isometric
drawing illustrating the
simplicity of the design
solution within the concept
of the site.

◁ Ground up projection
indicating the main
elements of the structure
and envelope to the
building.

91

Patient care areas occupy two of the wings. The layout of the treatment/consulting wing allows for clinical sessions in which patients may be seen in a consulting room individually and then join up with groups of patients in the health education area (e.g. antenatal sessions). It also allows for good staff communication between the treatment and consulting rooms. The consulting rooms can therefore be used as examination rooms as an extension of the treatment facility during clinic sessions. The chiropody and dental wing also contains a speech therapy suite. The main staff areas include a common room and should allow staff the opportunity of co-operation. Note the use of a separate kitchen and common room, allowing for access to the kitchen on those occasions when a staff meeting is taking place.

It is unfortunate that there was not the opportunity to integrate the adjacent GP with the centre to a greater extent. Nonetheless, the John Telford Clinic remains a useful lesson in sophistication and simplicity. This may well be due to the clarity of the brief and dialogue between the client group and the architects, but also to the ability of the architects rationally to assemble potentially conflicting and complex requirements into a coherent and flexible design solution. As with the Finsbury Health Centre, a sensitive design solution is achieved, essentially non-institutional yet not patronisingly domestic. It is a centre for health: invigorating, refreshing and uplifting.

Bridge Street Medical Centre

Location:	**Londonderry, Northern Ireland**
Completed:	**1989**
Type of facility:	**General practitioners' group practice premises**
Architects:	**Parker & Scott Architects**
Client:	**Dr T. Craig & Partners and Dr H. Leitch & Partners**
Gross floor area:	**465 sq m (5003 sq ft)**
Photography:	**Visuals Photography**

Architect's statement:

The medical centre was commissioned by six doctors from two separate practices, each with approximately 10,000 patients under their care.

Having acquired a derelict wasteland site the brief for the building was developed around the main criteria for accommodating two self-contained practices sharing waiting, reception and staff facilities. Each practice has three surgeries, a treatment room and records storage. A communal social worker's room is also provided.

Built in traditional building materials to marry with its neighbours, red facing brick and slated roof. The drama is provided by the use of deep soffets, large areas of glazing, corner buttressing and acute geometry.

The landscaped site provides the patients with adjacent car parking facilities, and a private doctors' car park.

Led by the brief to accommodate two practices with identical facilities the symmetrical plan evolved. Due to the specific needs of both the elderly and disabled patients, all treatment and consulting rooms are situated on the ground floor. Pressure from the local planning division to produce a building of two-storey height was contrary to the client's requirements and resulted in a deeply pitched roof offering useful space for staff quarters away from the view of patients.

The reception area allows patients views along

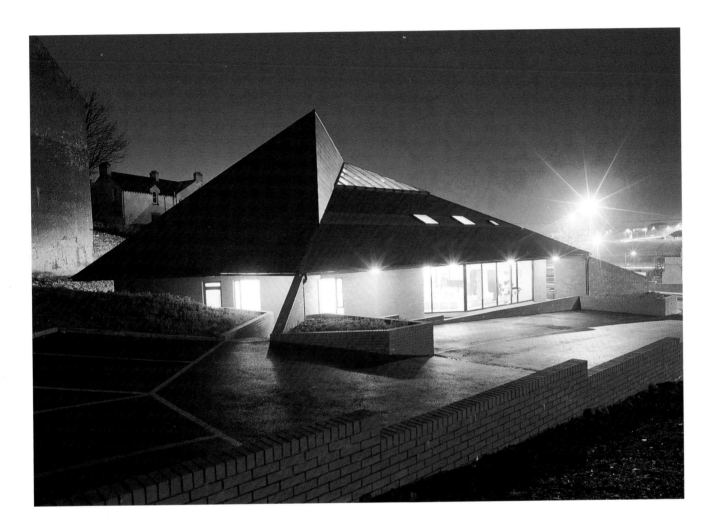

the River Foyle, whilst the apex roof glazing and first-floor void allows daylight to pass down through the centre of the building benefiting both first-floor staff areas and ground-floor reception station.

In 1989 the building won an RIBA regional award.

Main activity areas

Patient areas
Entrance lobby
Patient WCs
Waiting area
Treatment sub-wait (× 2)

Patient care areas
Social worker (interview)
GP Consulting room (× 6)
Treatment room (× 2)

Staff areas
Reception/records (× 2)
Library
Staff room
Shower/WC
Office (× 2)
Staff WC

△ *Bridge Street Medical Centre.*

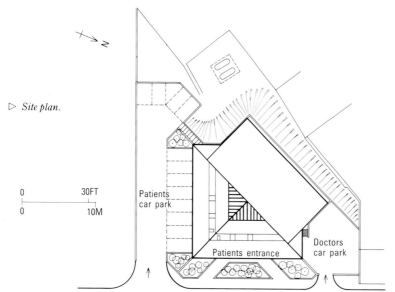

▷ *Site plan.*

0   30FT

0   10M

Comment

In contrast to the John Telford Clinic, the Bridge Street Medical Centre is a GP planned facility. It is the doctors themselves who identified the site under the financial package known as the 'Cost Rent Scheme'.

The site which remained derelict for 15 years was paradoxically owned by the local health authority. Dr Tom Craig and his two partners considered the site a good location for their new premises and began to negotiate with the health authority. However, it was over two years before

▷ *Ground-floor plan.*

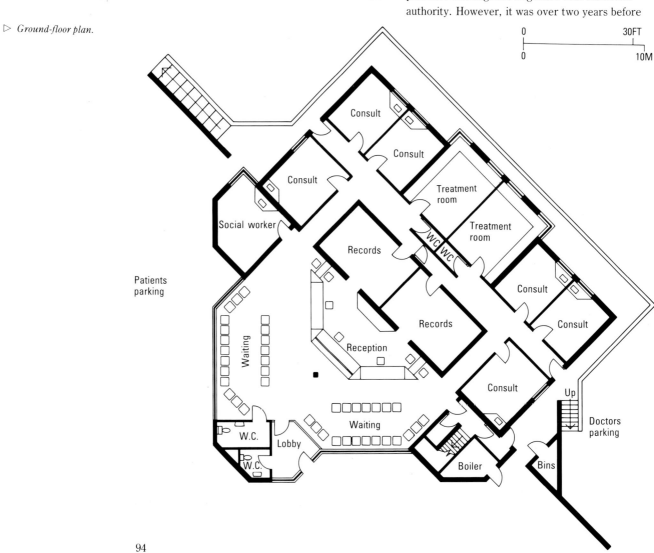

0   30FT

0   10M

94

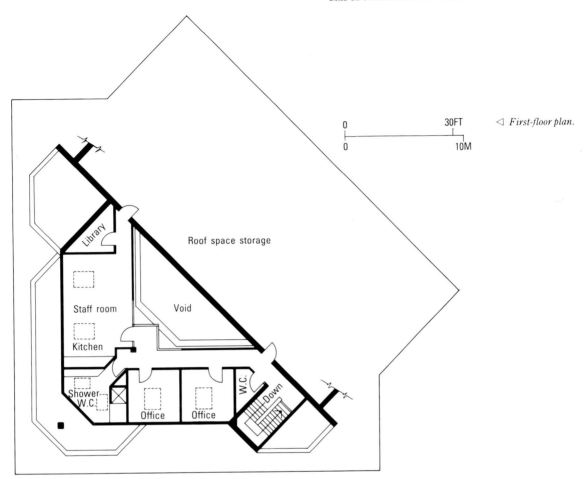

◁ *First-floor plan.*

an agreement could be reached, due to the health authority having first to consult with the Department of the Environment and Housing Executive as to whether they would require the land for their own use.

The involvement of the Central Services Agency (CSA – the equivalent of the FHSA) in the cost rent procedures brought the suggestion of teaming up with another group of doctors. The practice of Dr Leitch & Partners was also in need of better premises in the area. The CSA therefore played a positive and active role in bringing the two practices together to form an improved and more co-ordinated resource for primary health care for the local community.

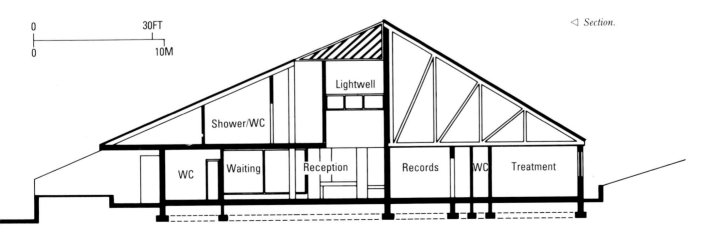

◁ *Section.*

▽ *View onto main entrance. The building's crisp and angular form brings relief to its rather nondescript surroundings.*

▽ *The reception working area benefits from a dramatic atrium pouring daylight into the central area of the building.*

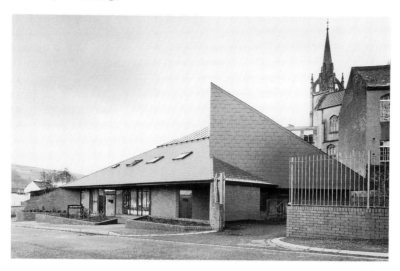

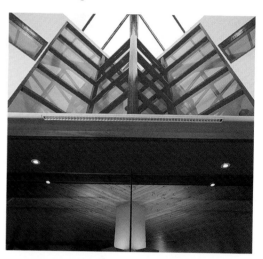

▷ *The reception area looking back to the main entrance. Note the lower level desk in the foreground enabling easier access for wheelchair users at reception.*

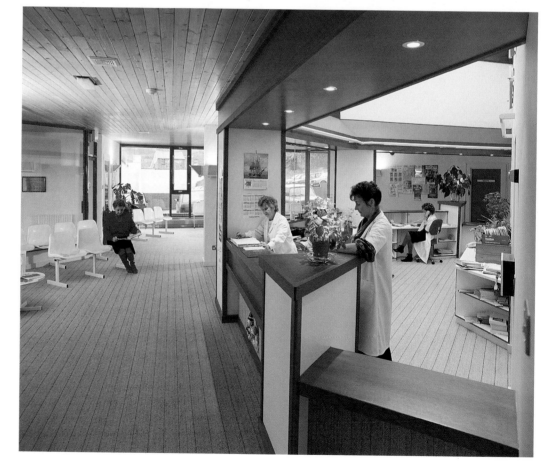

▽ *Staff corridor on the*
first floor looking into the
atrium space and down
into reception.

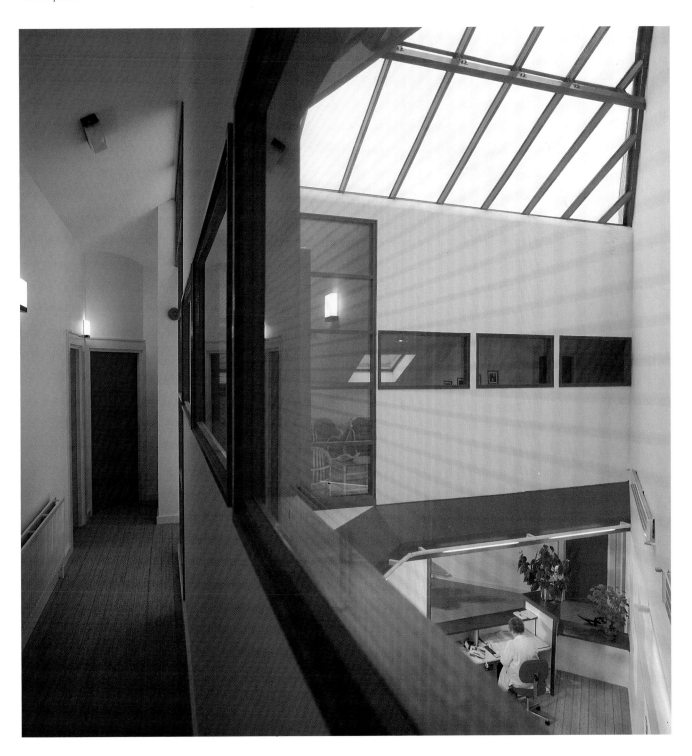

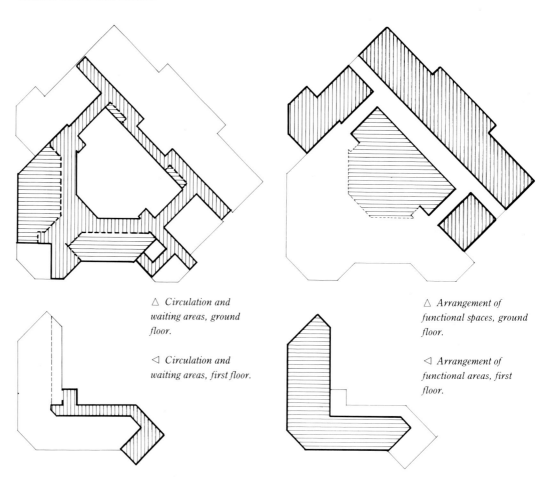

△ *Circulation and
waiting areas, ground
floor.*

◁ *Circulation and
waiting areas, first floor.*

△ *Arrangement of
functional spaces, ground
floor.*

◁ *Arrangement of
functional areas, first
floor.*

The symmetry of the plan is a clear reflection of
the combination of the two separate practices under
one roof.

From the main entrance the reception is well
positioned for visual supervision which extends to
the waiting area. The waiting area, although one
space, is divided into two seating areas, one for
each practice.

The reception desk includes two lower level
areas which can be used either by patients who
need to sit down, e.g. to complete a form, or by
wheelchair users. In considering the surroundings
of the locality the use of bright primary colours
seems appropriate. This, combined with the atrium
above the reception area, gives a feeling of
openness and informality.

From the waiting area patients pass to either side
of the reception desk to the patient care zone which
is in complete symmetry, and includes two WCs
associated with each treatment room. A door in the
middle of the patient care corridor completes the
joint use of space between the two practices.

The zoning of the plan allows staff to circulate
between staff and patient care areas discreetly,
without having to trespass into patient territory.
However, this is in part compromised by a sub-
waiting area for the treatment room in the patient
care corridor. An important criterion for the project
was to contain all patient contact areas on the
ground floor. The first floor is reserved exclusively
for staff use.

On the first floor both GP practices share the
staff room and library. Despite the symmetry of
separation in plan, the building functions as an
integrated facility. The practices are now becoming
more involved in screening and are able to offer a
wider range of services to their patients. The
building has therefore become an enabler for
primary health care.

The Bridge Street Medical Centre is an example
of an initially GP-led facility benefiting from the
intervention of the CSA in co-ordinating the
utilization of resources to provide improved primary
health care facilities.

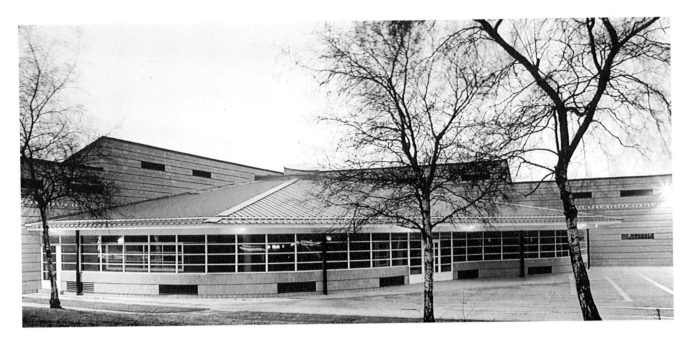

Lee Bank Health Centre

Location:	**Birmingham, The Midlands**
Completed:	**1988**
Type of facility:	**Health authority health centre**
Architects:	**Associated Architects**
Client:	**West Birmingham Health Authority**
Gross floor area:	**1100 sq m (11,836 sq ft)**
Photography:	**Alistair Carew-Cox**

Architect's statement:
Malcolm Booth and John Christophers
Associated Architects

The clients required a new health centre to service an inner city housing area built in the 1960s to the south west of Birmingham city centre. An existing doctors' practice operated from two converted maisonettes in an adjoining block of flats which was inadequate for the health care requirements of the area.

As well as consulting and treatment facilities for a practice of doctors, there was a need for dentistry, chiropody, physiotherapy, speech therapy, as well as maternity and social facilities.

There were no particular town planning constraints, the area having an amorphous, fragmented character and a wide mixture of building types. The planning officer and our clients were keen to have a building which had a very positive character of its own, both welcoming and friendly within the community.

The building site sits on a busy crossroads with multi-storey car parks on two corners and the damaged remnants of an 18th-century church on another.

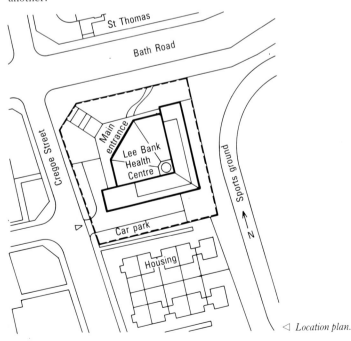

△ *The Lee Bank Health Centre, Birmingham.*

◁ *Location plan.*

▷ *The ground-floor plan combines the constraints of a formal structure of two wings accommodating the GP consulting and clinic facilities with a more informal waiting area, whose glass frontage floats beneath the roof, its informality a reflection of function.*

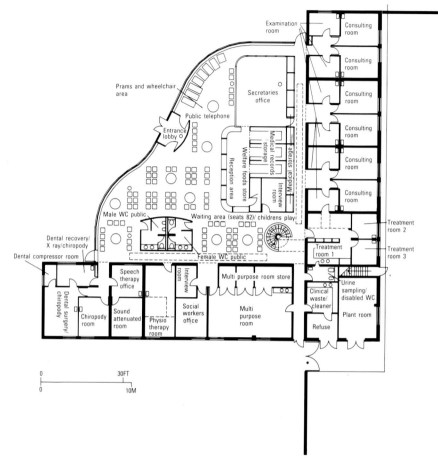

The centre was designed to face the crossroads on the diagonal with a fan shaped steel framed structure. This accommodates the entrance, reception and waiting spaces and enclosed on two sides by a one- and two-storey masonry structure containing the consulting and treatment rooms including all of the other support facilities.

The single-storey steel structure has a sandwich roof and an external curving glass wall of powder-coated steel glazing. The two-storey wings are clad in restructured stone-facing blocks with an artificial slate roof.

The road frontage remains open with access across a paved courtyard. The rear of the building is protected by a security fence to prevent unauthorised access to the consulting rooms and treatment rooms.

Comprehensive access for disabled people is provided.

The building was completed in 12 months to a very stringent budget, with funding partly from the Regional Health Authority and the Inner City Partnership.

Design concept

The design developed lies on a diagonal to the site, presenting its major frontage to the corner of Bath Road and Cregoe Street. There are two wings of professional and medical facilities surrounding and unified by a large open-plan public space.

The two wings contain the more static functions, with all consultation and medical facilities at ground floor, easily accessible yet screened where necessary from the patients' waiting area. The first-floor accommodation, which overlooks the ground floor waiting area, contains all those administrative and back-up facilities not requiring public access. Consequently, all parts of the

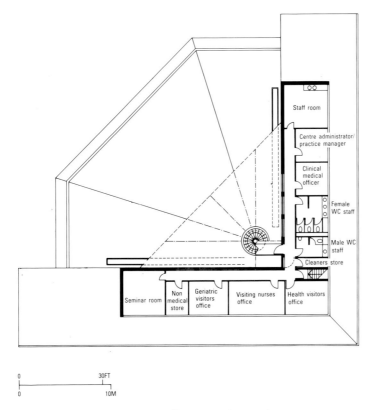

Staff room

Centre administrator/ practice manager

Clinical medical officer

Female WC staff

Male WC staff

Cleaners store

Seminar room | Non medical store | Geriatric visitors office | Visiting nurses office | Health visitors office

0 30FT

0 10M

building are closely related to each other.

The patients' waiting area, with its long span structure and use of free-standing modules of accommodation, provides an opportunity for future flexibility in use, along with the ability to break up waiting spaces into sub-groups located adjacent to their particular functions. The administration/ reception module forms a buffer between the main waiting area and the consulting rooms which are still within easy reach. The reception area is located to achieve command of the whole of the entrance and waiting areas.

With its presentation of a largely glazed public face to Bath Road and Cregoe Street, the building's security risks are minimized on the 'supermarket' principle of leaving the frontage open for easy surveillance. The back faces of the building are protected behind a security fence and being of masonry construction with small window openings can be protected against intruders.

Construction and structure

The building falls into two distinct structures: first the long span lightweight roofed waiting and reception area. This structure consists of circular concrete columns on individual concrete bases supporting open tubular steel lattice girder trusses radiating from a main column in the angle of the enclosed L-shaped block. The column is enveloped by the main spiral staircase to the first floor. This network of trusses supports the lattice steel purlins and a lightweight insulated metal deck roof. This roof is penetrated by a large circular roof-light over the main stair and by lighting slits abutting the wall of the two-storey block.

The external wall to this space is of sinuous curving glass, double-glazed with epoxy powder-coated metal frames. A low spandrel wall below the glazing forms a base for the heating and ventilation outlets. The free standing elements such as the

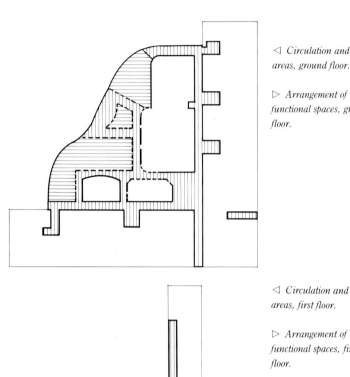

◁ *Circulation and waiting areas, ground floor.*

▷ *Arrangement of functional spaces, ground floor.*

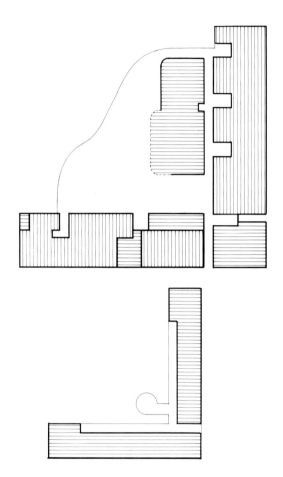

◁ *Circulation and waiting areas, first floor.*

▷ *Arrangement of functional spaces, first floor.*

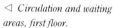

reception and secretary's area are completely independent of the structure.

The second structure is the short span two-storey heavy construction L-shaped block. Structurally separated from the long span roof to allow for differential movement this block houses all of the functions which are small span, cellular and which generally require a high degree of sound insulation and privacy. Consequently the construction is more traditional in its use of masonry block-faced cavity walls with internal partitions of dense concrete blocks, pre-cast concrete first floor and mono-pitched roofs of timber trussed rafters finished in slates.

The whole structure is built on a reinforced concrete raft to cope with the difficult ground conditions mentioned earlier.

Finishes

The L-shaped block has external walls finished in rusticated stone aggregate-faced concrete blocks designed to match the stonework of the church tower. All internal partitions are plaster finished. All windows are epoxy powder-coated steel and will not require repainting. All internal joinery is natural finish stained in various colours. Floors are generally finished with hard-wearing carpets, except in treatment rooms and other areas where non-slip finishes are required.

The roof of the L-shaped block is covered with dark blue-grey artificial slates. The long span roof is finished with a plastic coated self-coloured steel sheeting with matching steel gutters and rain-water pipes.

102

External works and landscaping

The building presents it public face on a diagonal to the corner of Cregoe Street and Bath Road with public access from both streets. Entry is down a short flight of steps or a ramp through landscaped banks of existing trees into a terrace paved in pre-cast concrete slabs divided up by strips of coloured concrete blocks. The landscaped banks are planted in low-maintenance ground cover and grass.

Vehicle access to the site is from Cregoe Street, the entrance protected by a barrier to prevent unauthorised parking. A large Tarmac surface car park and service area provides parking for 20 cars. Services access is through this car park for refuse removal and deliveries of medical supplies. A security fence and wall protect the service yard as well as the area to the east of the building containing consulting rooms.

The road frontages remain open. There is access to the main entrance for ambulances and disabled visitors. Disabled persons access into and around all public areas has been designed into the scheme.

Main activity areas

Patient areas
Entrance lobby, prams and wheelchair area
Waiting/children's play
Patient WC
Disabled specimen WC
Recovering (dental/chiropody/X-ray)

Patient care
Examination rooms (× 6)
Consulting rooms (× 6)
Treatment rooms (× 2)
Multi-purpose room
Interview rooms (× 2)
Physiotherapy room

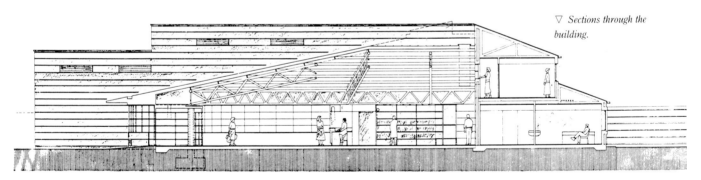

▽ *Sections through the building.*

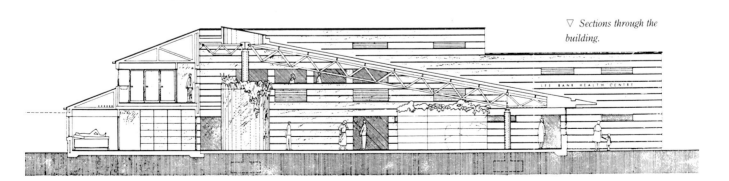

▽ *Sections through the building.*

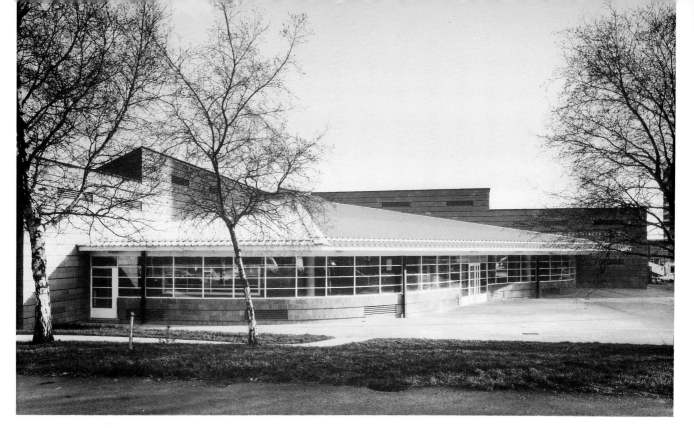

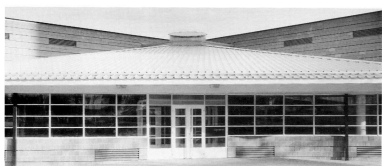

◁ *The glass wall facade was a deliberate open design taking account of security, based upon the supermarket principle of leaving a frontage open for ease of surveillance.*

△ *View on to main entrance.*

▷ *View on to the rear of clinic wing. Note the compatibility of the materials with the remains of the church in the background.*

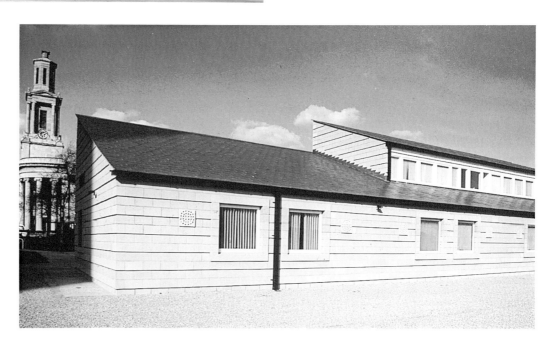

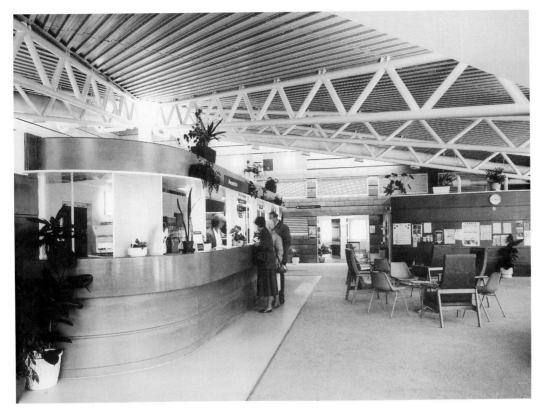

◁ *Reception/waiting area.*

▽ *Cut away axonometric looking onto the central waiting area.*

Sound attenuated room
Chiropody room
Dental surgery/chiropody

Staff areas
Social workers' office
Speech therapy office
Reception
Welfare food store
Medical store
Treatment utility
Medical records store
Secretary's office
Staff office
Centre administrator/practice manager
Clinical medical officer
Staff WCs
Health visitor's office
Visiting nurse office
Geriatric visitor's office
Seminar room

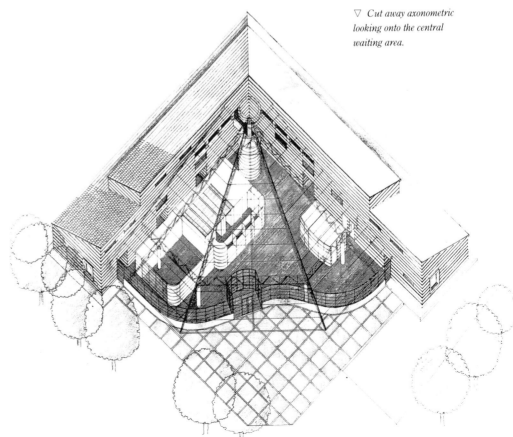

Comment

As with the John Telford Clinic, an essentially contemporary architectural aesthetic has been successfully harnessed to provide an appropriate environment for patient care. The building avoids any sense of institution without having to revert to the safety of a cosy domestic approach.

Entry to the reception desk does involve passing through the waiting area, but through use of screening, potential problems are averted.

As with the John Telford Clinic the pram shelter has been allocated a space inside the building and is visible from the reception and the majority of the waiting area.

In the GP consulting wing (in contrast to the Bridge Street Medical Centre) each doctor has in addition to a consulting room separate examination rooms. This may be a reflection of the different funding arrangements. At Lee Bank the GPs were not involved in the financing of the project. If GPs undertake examinations in their consulting rooms the necessary level of examination room provision would be in excess of the recommendations of available research with regard to the utilization of consulting suites. One of the examination rooms also has two doors. This potentially restricts the amount of usable space and could compromise confidentiality.

The treatment suite merits special attention. Working closely with the client, the architects recognized that there are two fundamental activities associated with treatment:

- Patient care for examinations, etc.
- Utility storage and analysis of materials.

This was taken into account in the design – the Lee Bank treatment suite is arranged so that staff may enter the space and obtain materials without having to walk through the area where a patient may be being examined. Additionally the two treatment rooms are properly separated by a partition rather than merely a curtain as seen in earlier health centres. The location of a specimen WC also allows for the discreet transfer of a sample from the WC through to the treatment room for collection and/or analysis.

The second wing of the centre contains a large multi-purpose room which is used for health education involving group sessions, fulfilling the recognized need for greater emphasis for opportunities for preventive medicine.

As with the Bridge Street Medical Centre, all patient contact areas have been contained on the ground floor with the first floor accommodating staff only. A further aid to staff co-operation is provided in the form of a seminar room, in addition to the staff room.

Lee Bank embodies many of the fundamental principles of a primary health care building. Within one shell a whole range of medical practitioners have the opportunity of working together to create an integrated team approach to primary care.

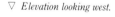
▽ *Elevation looking west.*

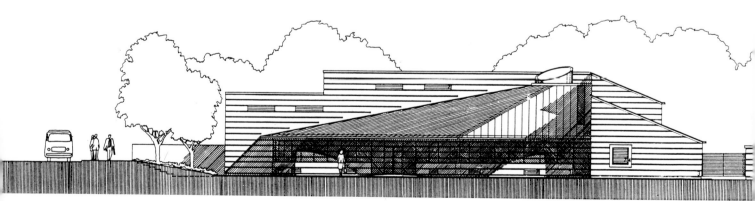

Highgate Group Practice

Location:	**Highgate, London**
Completed:	**1986**
Type of facility:	**General practitioners' group practice premises**
Architects:	**Douglas Stephen & Partners**
Client:	**The Highgate Group Practice (co-ordinators Dr S. Dukes, Dr C. Hindley and Dr L. Rose)**
Gross floor area:	**544 sq m (5853 sq ft)**
Photography:	**Martin Charles**

Architect's statement:
Stephen Gage, Douglas Stephen & Partners

The Highgate Group Practice building is located in North Hill, Highgate, London, an area which typifies the historic accretions found in most British towns and cities. The overall impression is that of a North American Main Street put together over 500 rather than 50 years. The neighbourhood contains a bit of everything from the elegance of Tectons Highpoint (the same architects designed Finsbury Health Centre) to the 18th-century cottages opposite.

The proposed site for the health centre was inauspicious. The houses built recently to the south are set well back from the road and face a central courtyard. The rear gardens which front on to the road are not considered as a suitable form to respond to, but rather to react against.

In developing the forms of this building I attempted to make them as simple, direct and appropriate as possible, since each step had to be discussed with eight clients (i.e. members of the Highgate Group Practice). The choice of finishes – pale bricks, steel, glass, white plaster and carpet – had to pass the scrutiny of both clients and local people. This tended to support the rationalist abstraction of detail because the process became one of exclusion whereby only familiar, simple, well-liked materials remained part of the scheme. There was also a clear definition of elements that

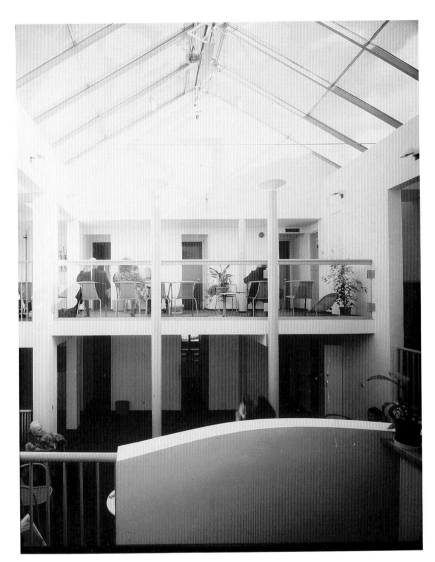

△ *Highgate Group Practice.*

were forbidden. For example, it was most pleasing to be asked to design a medical building without a significant corridor or a main signboard. Moreover, no references to current hospital design were allowed.

Most medical buildings are either based on lifts and corridors or are grossly extended single-storey buildings. There was a strong feeling on the part of the clients that their building should break the mould. The doctors took two crucial decisions: they chose to leave their consulting rooms to examine wheelchair patients in a room which was part of the

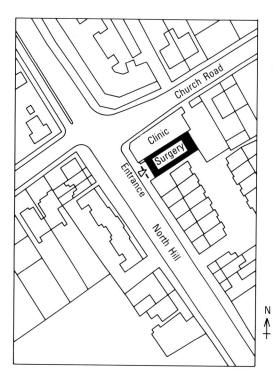

▷ *Location plan.*

main treatment complex at the front of the building. This allowed generous stair circulation in the main courtyard of the building with an atrium-type space instead of the more usual lift/corridor type of plan. They also chose to have one entrance to the building. A separate staff passageway was rejected and replaced by *en suite* rooms on either side of the entrance hall.

During the design process I realized that in this building I was constructing not one reality but a series of interlocking worlds. At all stages the primary consideration was to create a therapeutic journey for the patients. In a sense doctors are 'on stage' when 'on duty'.

When the administrative staff are treated, like the doctors and nurses, as part of the operation of the building, the on stage/off stage analogy applies equally to them. The function of the staff room in this building is complex. It can be considered as a 'green room' where staff can meet offstage, but it is also a room where strategy is planned. It opens on to two flat roofs where staff can sit in fine weather.

▷ *Ground-floor plan. The layout follows a logical progression from entry through to reception and then waiting. Access to all consulting rooms requires the negotiation of at least one flight of stairs. However, for disabled or physically frail patients doctors undertake the consultation in the ground-floor treatment suite.*

▷ *First-floor plan. Apart from the upper-level suite of four consulting rooms the first floor comprises staff use areas accessed off the entrance hall. These enjoy side balcony areas and a sense of external space.*

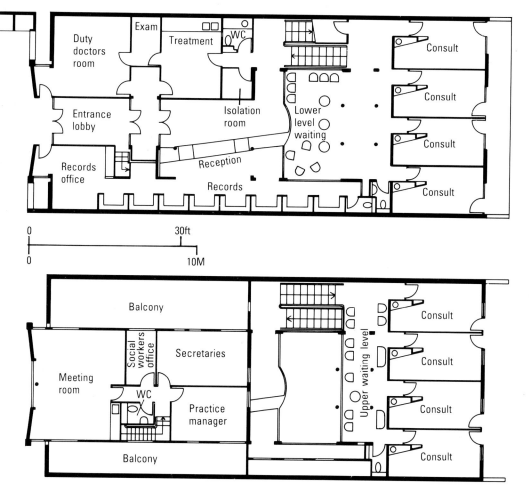

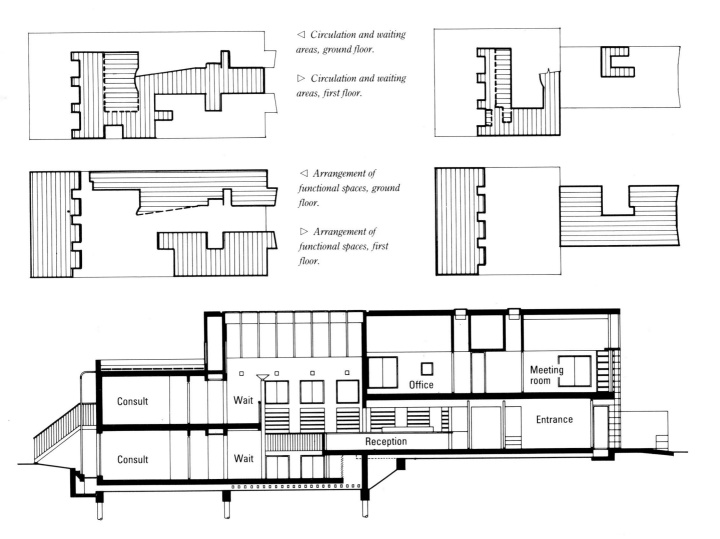

◁ Circulation and waiting areas, ground floor.

▷ Circulation and waiting areas, first floor.

◁ Arrangement of functional spaces, ground floor.

▷ Arrangement of functional spaces, first floor.

Consult

Wait

Consult

Wait

Office

Meeting room

Reception

Entrance

△ Cross-section.

The most important space in the building is the central courtyard. It acts as an external facade to a building which is severely limited by its site boundaries on both sides and therefore required lighting mainly from above. Its external quality is, in part, its origin as the point where all different worlds in the building meet.

Front of house and meeting room

The patient's first contact with the clinic is at the reception desk. The staff behind it control and process the records of 18,000 patients. This work is frequently hidden away, however the clients wanted the administrative staff to be a visible part of the operation of the building. The central treatment room of the practice (part of an examination/treatment suite) is occupied by the practice nurse.

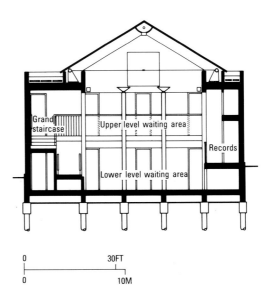

Grand staircase

Upper level waiting area

Records

Lower level waiting area

| 0 | 30FT |
| 0 | 10M |

◁ Long section.

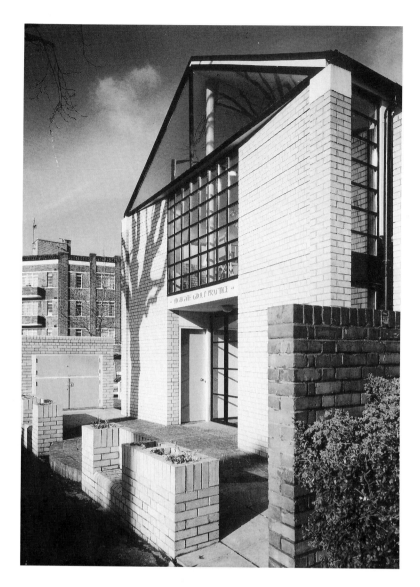

△ *View to main entrance. First-floor window and glazing above is the staff room.*

▷ *Waiting areas to lower and upper levels contained within an informal atrium space. Despite the building's essentially contemporary aesthetic, the centre has a feel not dissimilar to that of an English country house.*

Main activity areas

Patients
Entrance hall
Waiting area (× 2)
Patient WCs
Specimen WCs

Patient care
Consulting rooms (× 8)
Shared examination room (× 2)
Treatment room/duty doctor's room

Staff
Reception
Records area and processing
Secretary's office
Practice administration
Social worker's office
Meeting room
Staff WCs

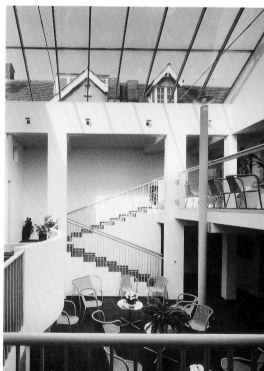

The patient's journey starts at a clearly defined entrance which leads past the reception desk to a main glazed court. A separate waiting area leads to the treatment rooms. The main courtyard – the waiting room – is on two levels, the upper with a balcony looking onto the main space. Although the doctors have a sophisticated communication system they choose to invite patients into their consulting room personally.

The eight consulting rooms each have an ante-chamber facing the main space, as well as a stair to the car park and garden area at the rear of the site. The steel frame supporting the balcony and the main roof distinguishes the separate waiting areas from the circulation paths.[1]

Comment

In contrast to the Bridge Street Medical Centre where two separate practices are 'married' by circumstance, the Highgate Group Practice was already an established eight doctor practice. It had a local reputation as a caring and forward group of doctors. They had previously practised in a Victorian house nearby. Having put up with the fact that an inappropriate building can restrict and often frustrate the workings of a busy practice, the doctors came to the briefing process determined that their new building would not do the same.

Within a highly restrictive site the design of the Highgate Group Practice breaks almost all the rules, yet works. The solution is every bit a result of a particularly articulate client as an inventive architect.

From entry the circulation route leads directly to the reception desk. Visitors are therefore able to make appointments, collect prescription notes or make general enquiries without the need to penetrate the building any further (such visitors can account for 30% of users).

From reception the building divides into an upper and lower level with the exception of the treatment suite. Patients therefore have to negotiate at least one flight of stairs to see their doctor. However, the ground-floor treatment suite is available 'for use by those patients who would be unable to use the stairs'. This of course relies upon the doctors undertaking to walk out of their consulting rooms to the treatment area (something they are willing to do and as this was brought into the design brief).

The two waiting areas may still be compromised in terms of privacy for waiting patients. It is possible for those waiting to observe patients and staff enter and leave the consulting rooms. Whilst it is understood that the staff would not mind being on view to waiting patients, the patients have little choice but to be a part of the building's informality.

On the other hand, this arrangement allows the doctors to continue as in their previous surgery – to call their patients personally and not rely upon a call system. The doctors would come out of their rooms, greet their patients at the door and welcome them into their consulting room. It could be argued that this more informal and personal approach can balance the disadvantage of patients waiting outside the consulting room. The

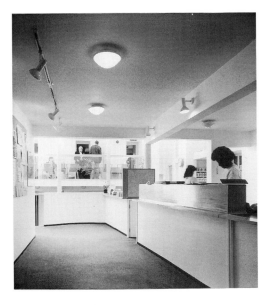

◁ *The reception desk, clearly visible from point of entry, can be located without having to negotiate the waiting area.*

▽ *Staff room looking out on to the main entrance.*

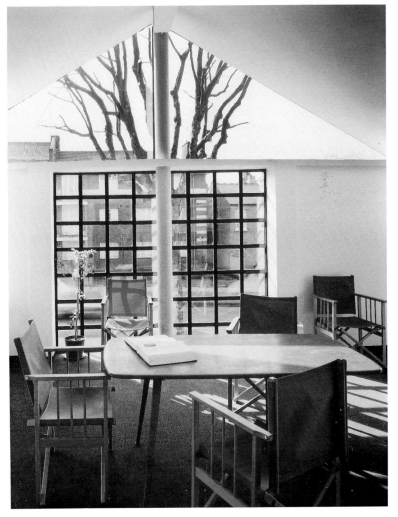

111

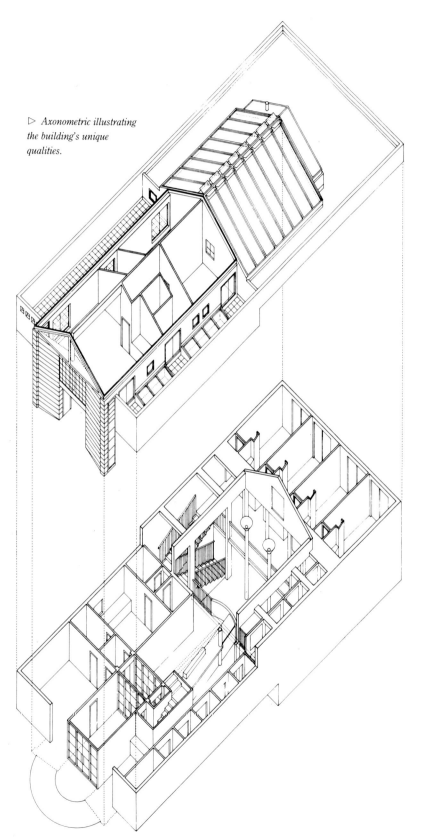

▷ *Axonometric illustrating the building's unique qualities.*

arrangement of the waiting area to the consulting rooms is permanent, whereas the policy of the doctors coming out to greet the patients could (in theory) be made redundant by a future management regime.

Restrictive width of the site has no doubt forced the compromise of the corridor through the rooms of the treatment suite. Here there are three rooms:

- Treatment room
- Shared examination room
- Duty doctor's office

Having accepted the use of levels to provide the required floor space, the internal spaces which they create offer a most calming and informal place in which to visit and work. The design of the consulting rooms, which have integrated the activity of examination via an alcove, is a discreet solution, allowing both consulting and examination to take place within one cellular room.

Although there is no area specifically designed for patient group activities, the meeting space on the first floor is available as such. It is difficult to do justice to this building by simply studying the plan. One can begin to understand its true sense of space by the architect's axonometric drawings.

The Highgate Group Practice fits around the philosophy and requirements of a particular client. The building will, however, inevitably outlive the working lifespan of its original client and new occupants will have to work within the philosophy laid down by their forebears. If the philosophy is sound then this can be viewed as a positive device to ensure that any desire for a move away from the them/patients and us/doctors imagery will live on.

Reference

1. *AA File*, No. 13 (Autumn 1986).

Manor Place Surgery

Location:	**Walworth Road, South London**
Completed:	**1991**
Type of facility:	**General practitioners' group practice premises**
Architect:	**Penoyre & Prasad**
Client:	**Drs Higgs, Haigh, McKay and Rayburn**
Gross floor area:	**507 sq m (5455 sq ft)**

Architect's statement:
Gregory Penoyre

This is a busy and expanding doctors' practice which has been working in cramped conditions in a shop unit and house in 206 Walworth Road. Searches were made for a suitable alternative site on which to develop a new practice. After extensive research no suitable site was available. Because the position of the present practice is ideal for patients, a site linked to the rear of the present practice was purchased for development. This comprised of a long thin builder's yard and a three-storey building on the adjoining Manor Place.

The design

The new surgery provides a seven doctor unit. This consists of a refurbished original building at 206 Walworth Road linked to a new two-storey wing built in the yard at the rear of 1 Manor Place. The site is enclosed by other properties to the west of the two-storey buildings and to the north and east by the back of shops and flats on Walworth Road and Manor Place.

The new surgery is entered from Manor Place through an existing archway leading to the main reception and waiting areas in the new part of the building. There are waiting areas distributed to reception and office. Because ground-floor space

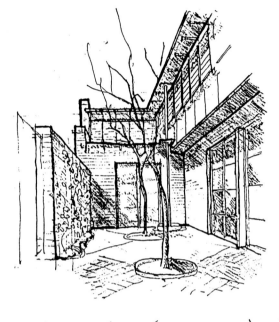

◁ Manor Place Surgery, London. View to courtyard.

▽ Location plan.

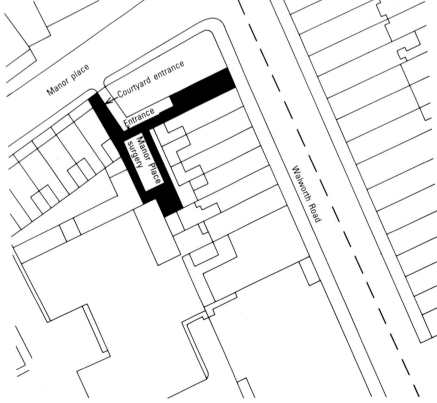

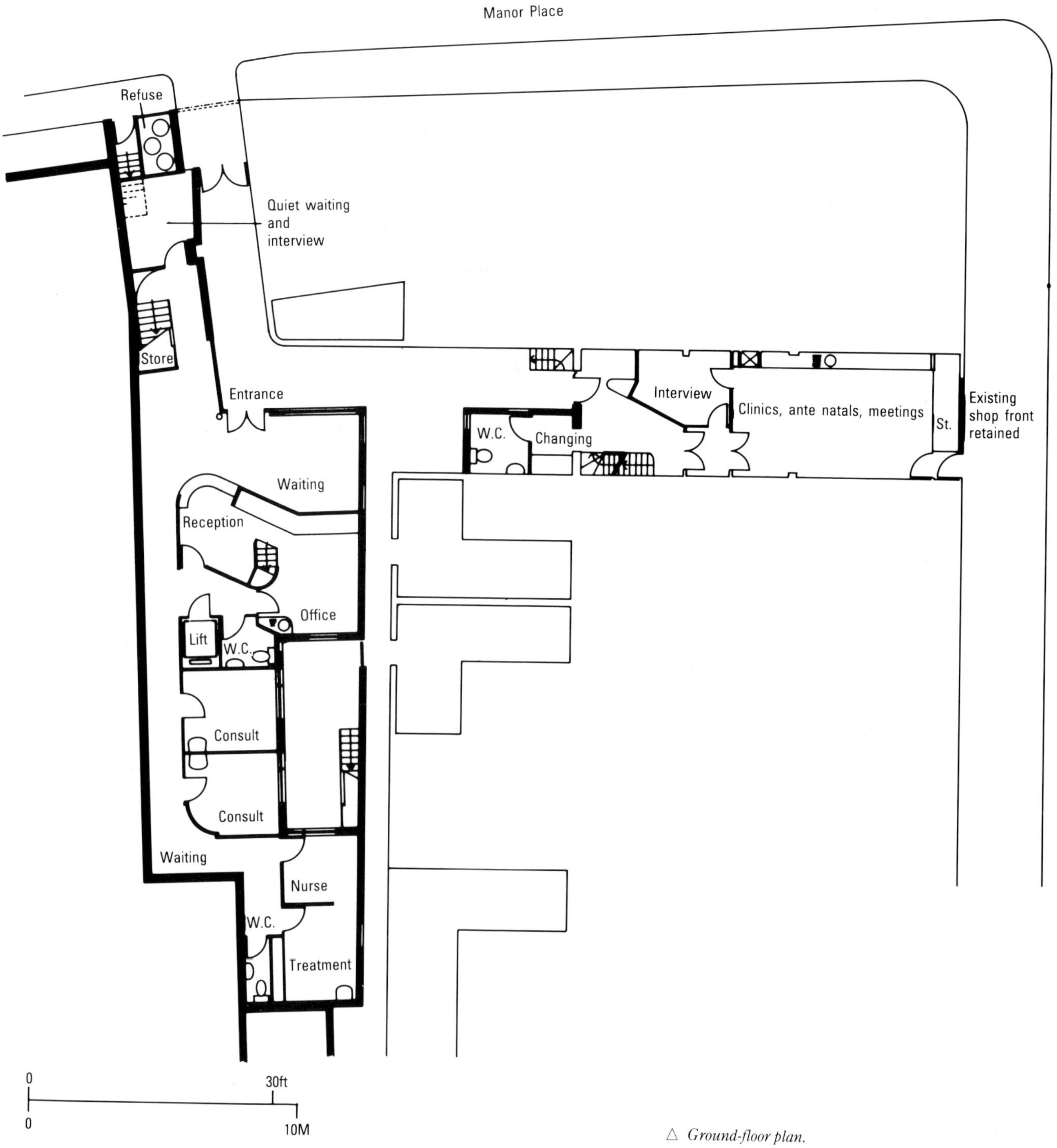

Manor Place

Refuse

Quiet waiting
and
interview

Store

Entrance

Interview

Clinics, ante natals, meetings

St.

Existing
shop front
retained

W.C.

Changing

Waiting

Reception

Office

Lift

W.C.

Consult

Consult

Waiting

Nurse

W.C.

Treatment

Walworth Road

0

30ft

0

10M

△ *Ground-floor plan.*

114

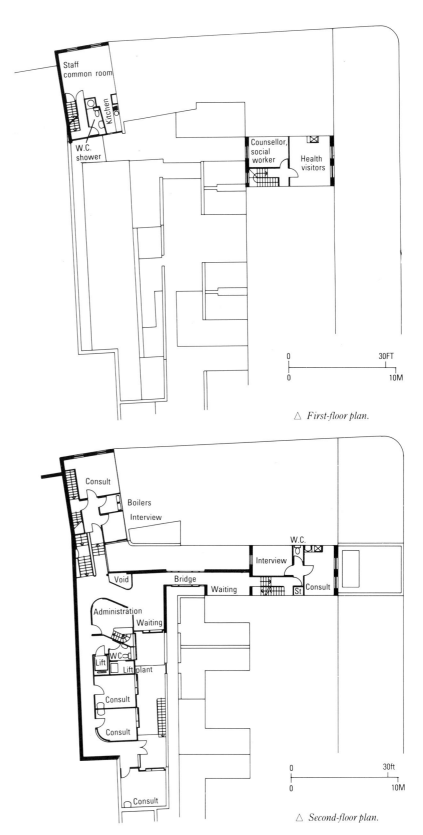

was at a premium it was necessary to place two consulting rooms and the treatment room on the ground floor and the remaining five consulting rooms on the first. Consequently a small lift is provided adjacent to the reception area to allow wheelchairs and patients of limited mobility access to the first floor. On the first floor there are also interview rooms and an administration office that overlooks the upper waiting room. Staff offices and other facilities are placed on the second floor of the two existing buildings. At ground level there is also a secondary entrance at the rear of 206 Walworth Road allowing part of the premises to be used separately and at times when the surgeries are closed. This leads to a multi-purpose space for group activities: health education, clinics and health promotion uses.

An existing right of way had to be maintained at all times running from Manor Place to the rear of the properties on the Walworth Road necessitating a bridge at first-floor level from the new part of the building to the consulting and interview rooms and to the other facilities in 206 Walworth Road. Specific provision has also been made to deal with security from users of the right of way and refuse produced by them and the surgery.

The form of the new building has been designed with particular concern for the problems of daylighting, overlooking and privacy. The ground floor has been arranged so that the two consulting rooms, the treatment room and the office on the ground floor open on to a small garden court. This has a high perforated garden wall and trellis between it and the right of way that runs along the backs of the adjacent properties on Walworth Road, preventing viewing from these properties. On the first floor the building steps back on either side to allow light into the courtyard below and so as not to over-shadow adjoining properties. Overlooking is also avoided on the first floor by reducing the size of the windows facing on to the courtyard and neighbouring buildings by use of deep projecting eaves. The consequent loss of light is regained by a roof-lighting at the back of these rooms at the top of a curved, lightweight aluminium roof.

△ *First-floor plan.*

△ *Second-floor plan.*

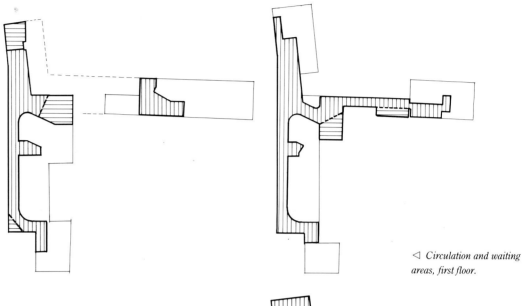

▷ *Circulation and waiting areas, ground floor.*

◁ *Circulation and waiting areas, first floor.*

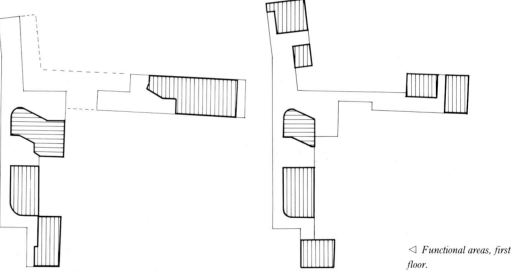

▷ *Functional areas, ground floor.*

◁ *Functional areas, first floor.*

The new building is constructed in load-bearing brick and block to first-floor level forming a base and lighter timber frame ply clad external walls to the courtyard from first floor to roof. There are dense concrete block internal partitions and concrete first-floor slabs for acoustic separation. Windows are timber with steel opening lights. Flat roof terraces are 'upside down' asphalt roof with paving. The curved sloping section of roof over the main part is profiled aluminium on timber rafters.

Main activity areas

Patients
Waiting area (× 4)
Quiet waiting
WCs
Specimen WCs
Patient changing

116

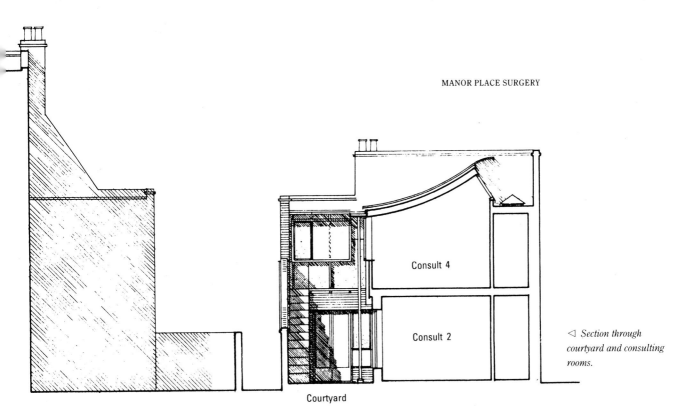

Consult 4

Consult 2

Courtyard

◁ *Section through
courtyard and consulting
rooms.*

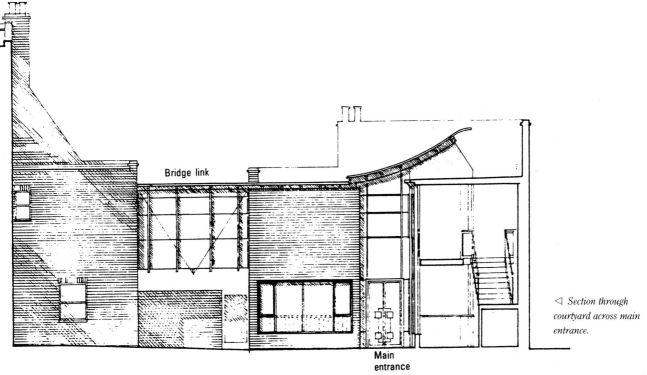

Bridge link

Main
entrance

◁ *Section through
courtyard across main
entrance.*

Patient care

Consulting rooms (× 7)
Treatment/Nurse
Interview (× 4)*
Group space/multi-purpose

* Room with dual function of waiting and interview.

Staff

Reception
Office
Administration
Staff common room
Kitchen
WC/shower

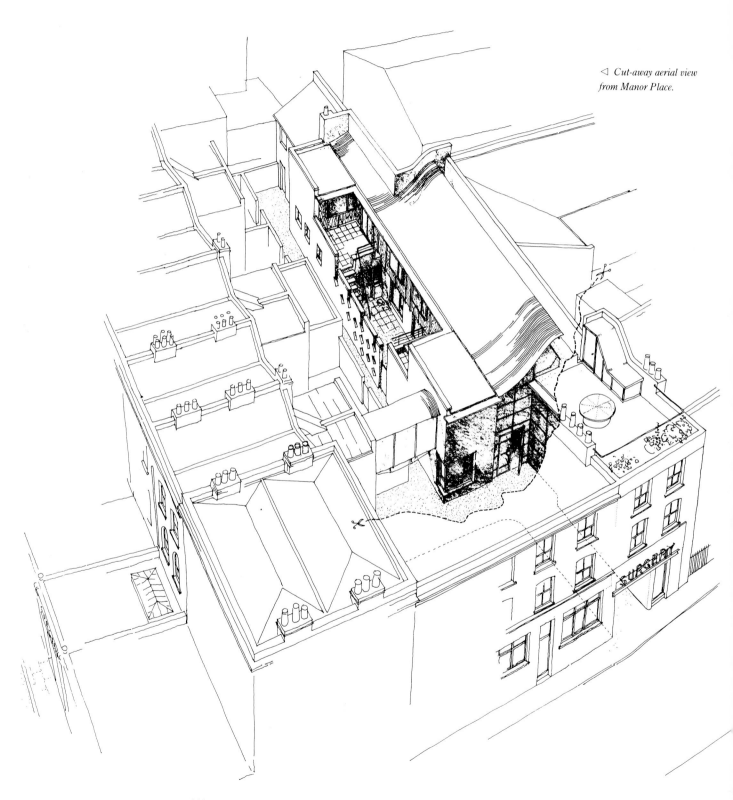

◁ *Cut-away aerial view
from Manor Place.*

Comment

Because primary health care centres, by their very
nature, should be easily accessible to the local
community, the possibility of purpose-built facilities
will not always be possible. The Highgate Group
Practice managed to overcome the constraints of a
typical urban infill site. Manor Place presented the
architects with the constraints of having to work
within an existing shell on a highly complex site.

The search for a suitable site can often represent
the longest period in the lifespan of a primary health
care project. Even when the location is identified,
its price is often prohibitive as it will need to
compete with the potential site value for more
commercial projects. Land values in such instances
can place the proportion of building costs as a
comparatively small percentage compared with that
of the overall project costs.

At Manor Place as at Highgate, the project
became an exercise in ensuring that the expensive
resource of space would be used effectively and
efficiently.

From Manor Place the entrance is approached via
an enclosed passageway. From reception, patients
either wait by the first waiting area or are directed
elsewhere. The ground floor contains two
consulting rooms and the treatment suite, each
looking on to an internal courtyard. The sub-waiting
area for the treatment rooms is accommodated
within the circulation route (as is the waiting area
for consulting room 7 and the associated interview
room).

It is important to be able to segregate patients
who will be visiting the centre for different kinds of
sessions, however, privacy may be compromised
outside these rooms, particularly on the ground
floor.

The arrangement of the multi-purpose group
space (which may also be accessed off Walworth
Road) allowed for a number of possibilities. Its shop
front facade can promote health education as a
walk-in self-contained facility, further breaking
away from the image of an institution. Whilst it is
separate at ground level it becomes linked with the
rest of the centre at first floor. The group space
can therefore be perceived as separate from the
doctors' surgery yet benefiting from the input of
the surgery activities, and vice versa.

The introduction of a lift allows patients to use
the first floor, therefore the capital investment is
justified by a greater area of usable space for
patient care. The route from the lift to the first-
floor waiting area and back to the consulting rooms
does not contain the inherent logic of a purpose-
built facility. It would have been preferable for
patients to be able visually to locate the first-floor
waiting area upon arrival from the lift. However,
there is an advantage in that staff can circulate
discreetly from the lift to reception and
administration on the first floor.

It is worth noting that of the patient care areas
nine out of 13 (70%) may be accessed without a
patient having to use stairs. Only consulting rooms
6 and 7, together with their adjacent interview
rooms, provide a rather lengthy route for both
patients and staff. Yet this must be accepted as part
of the inevitable compromise that the restraints of
an existing building involve.

Manor Place Surgery has many of the qualities of
the Highgate Group Practice. It is an example of a
scheme in which an architect has worked very
closely with an informed and highly articulate client,
and has therefore been able to craft a rather
sophisticated design solution out of a constrained
site.

The tension between functional criteria and this
restrictive site has been transformed into a dynamic
use of light and space. The quality of the Manor
Place Surgery design far exceeds many purpose-
built schemes which have none of the complexities
of this site to contend with.

The Crowndale Health Centre

Location:	**Camden Town, North London**
Completed:	**1989**
Type of facility:	**Integrated primary health care centre including clinic, dental and doctor's surgery**
Architect:	**Rock Townsend**
Client:	**London Borough of Camden and the Bloomsbury Health Authority**
Gross floor area:	**1965 sq m (21,000 sq ft)**
	Part of a larger community complex of 10,737 sq m (116,000 sq ft)

Architect's statement:
Wendy Mason, Project Architect, Rock Townsend

In 1984 the London Borough of Camden declared Camden Town a 'priority area'. It recognized, after long campaigning by the local community, that the southern half of the area (Sommerstown in particular) suffered from a fragmented health and housing repair service.

▽ *Location plan. The Crowndale Health Centre is part of a community resource facility including social, housing services plus workshop, retail and office space with a cafe all under one roof.*

A large post office building came on the market in the autumn of 1985. Rock Townsend Architects were commissioned to carry out a feasibility study which concluded that the site was ideal for the development of a multi-service centre which would address local needs. The London Borough of Camden bought the building in March 1986 on one of the last sale and lease-back transactions before the Government deemed this method illegal.

The Bloomsbury Health Authority in a unique partnership with the local authority bought their own position within the centre and paid Camden for a new building.

Briefing began in earnest in the spring of 1986 and the design was completed ready for construction on site in October 1987. The construction included specialist fitting out and was completed in the autumn of 1989. The health centre was officially opened in December 1989.

The facilities

The health centre offers the following services to the community:

- Child health clinics for babies up to five
- Antenatal classes and clinics for expectant mothers
- Dental and orthodontic clinics for children
- Speech therapy for children
- Family planning clinics
- General Practitioner surgery
- Chiropody clinics
- Treatment room for minor ailments, dressing, injections, etc.
- Base for community psychiatric nurses

The centre also includes generous facilities for health education, the emphasis being on preventive medicine rather than cure.

Philosophy

The brief for the health centre was a complex jigsaw puzzle of well-defined specialist functions

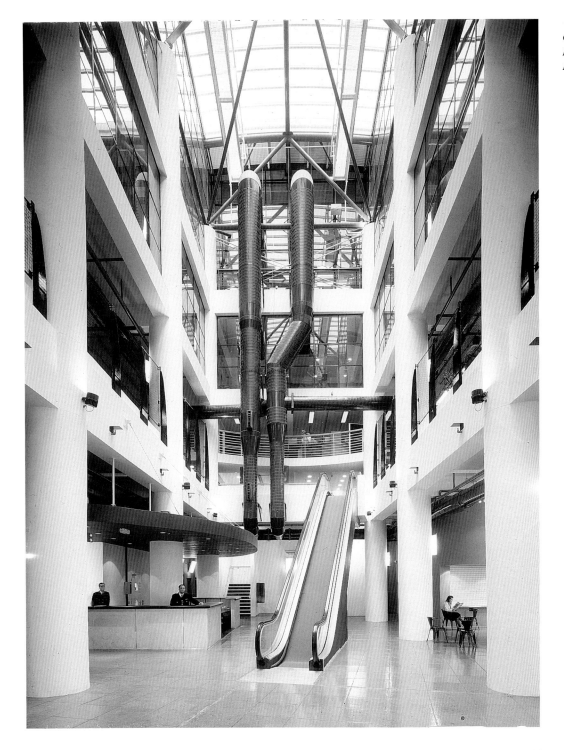

◁ *Crowndale Health*
Centre, Camden Town,
London. Photography:
Peter Cook.

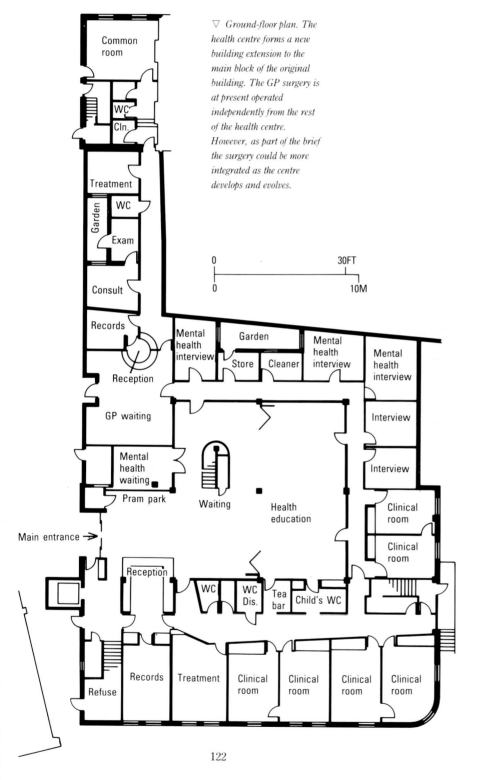

▽ *Ground-floor plan. The health centre forms a new building extension to the main block of the original building. The GP surgery is at present operated independently from the rest of the health centre. However, as part of the brief the surgery could be more integrated as the centre develops and evolves.*

Common room

WC

Cln.

Treatment

Garden

WC

Exam

Consult

Records

Reception

GP waiting

Mental health interview

Garden

Store   Cleaner

Mental health interview

Mental health interview

Interview

Mental health waiting

Pram park

Waiting

Health education

Interview

Clinical room

Clinical room

Main entrance →

Reception

WC

WC Dis.

Tea bar

Child's WC

Refuse

Records

Treatment

Clinical room

Clinical room

Clinical room

Clinical room

0 ────────── 30FT
0 ────────── 10M

with specific relationships. It required good natural light, privacy, accessibility and clear circulation patterns. It became clear at an early stage that the existing main building with its general floor-to-ceiling height and deep plan did not lend itself to the more intimate character required for the health centre. We therefore decided that it was necessary to design a new facility to the rear of the main building which would then accommodate the health centre.

The philosophy from the outset was to create a fully integrated centre offering a range of services to the community under one roof – housing, social services, planning consultations, etc. as well as the services of a primary health care facility. A balance was needed between allowing the health centre a certain amount of autonomy whilst avoiding isolating it altogether. This was achieved by making the main entrance to the centre highly visible from both the street (from the Crowndale Road alleyway) and the 'public square' on the ground floor of the main building. The latter is not dominated by the functional requirements of the London Borough of Camden, and care has been taken by all to avoid creating a mini Town Hall. It houses a public cafe, retail units, exhibition space and an information desk. It also gives access to all the centre's facilities, including of course the health centre.

Spatial arrangements

The massing of the new health centre building was determined by a number of factors. Economic pressures demanded that both the London Borough of Camden and the Bloomsbury Health Authority build a commercially viable building, therefore the maximum possible floor area was required on the site as a whole. This necessitated building to house office accommodation for both the Bloomsbury Health Authority as well as space to let. Privacy and light consideration for adjoining building owners dictated the position of the four-storey structure. The brief required easy accessibility and therefore ground-floor accommodation was in high demand. To achieve this we filled in the residual site up to and including the end terraced house off Crowndale Road with a single-storey structure.

The four-storey structure is an *in situ* concrete flat slab structure with rendered block cavity wall and coloured steel windows. The steel framed curved roof hovers over the whole and echoes the larger version on the main building. The single storey consists of load-bearing cavity walls, steel and timber structure, with an upside-down flat roof finish. The 'conservatory' roof is in aluminium patent glazing.

Externally, the simple white rendered elevations have been treated differently to reflect the changes in plan and elevation at each level. The ground floor of the existing terraced house (now part of the GP accommodation), the long single-storey walls and the four-storey structure have been visually linked by a continuous band of rusticated render. The restrictions are repeated on the ground floor of the main building where it faces the health centre in the alleyway from Crowndale Road. The latter space terminates dramatically at the lift tower at the intersection of the two blocks, beneath which is the entrance to the health centre and the public square of the main building. The formal relationship between the two buildings is further strengthened by the two curved walls and windows (similar both in colour and type) in both brick and rendered wall.

The ground floor has a 'central square' as its main focus, containing the waiting area and main health education space with flexible screening for sub-division if required. This focus is the most public part of the building and is directly accessible from the entrance. It is half set within the four-storey building and half without. The latter half is top-lit via a conservatory which links the public waiting area of the dental suite at first floor to the main space below.

The central space is bounded on three sides by a semi-private translucent glazed cloister which gives direct access to the consulting rooms which are arranged around the perimeter of the building where they take advantage of natural light and ventilation. This arrangement has enabled us to handle the move from public to semi-private to very private space with sensitivity. It also establishes a legible circulation system which avoids the plethora of corridors and dead-ends traditionally found in health buildings.

The detail, colour and materials have been chosen to create a bright, welcoming atmosphere without sacrificing functional and hygiene standards. The main public area is bright and well lit with a warm beech floor. Intimacy is achieved at the reception desk by a coloured drop bulk head. The internal corridor to the suite of rooms on the ground floor has splayed walls, large round columns and colours which convey quiet and privacy. The highly serviced elements of the individual consulting rooms have been arranged together at one end, leaving the main space naturally lit with possible flexibility of layout – location of couch, desk, chairs, etc. These simple but bright spaces are strong enough visually to control the inevitable mix of furniture and instruments whose choice will inevitably be left to others.

▽ *First-floor plan. Further accommodation to include a mental health waiting area and meeting room is located on the third floor. The second-floor and the remainder of the third-floor accommodation is for offices to be used by Bloomsbury Health Authority and to be let to outside users.*

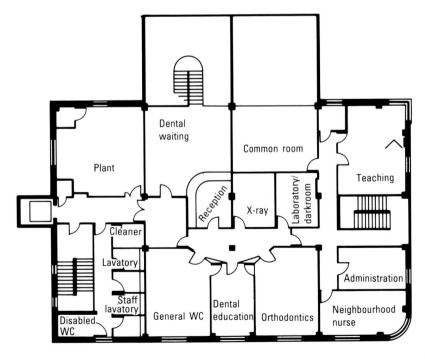

▷ *Circulation and waiting areas, first floor.*

▷ *Staff and patient care areas, first floor.*

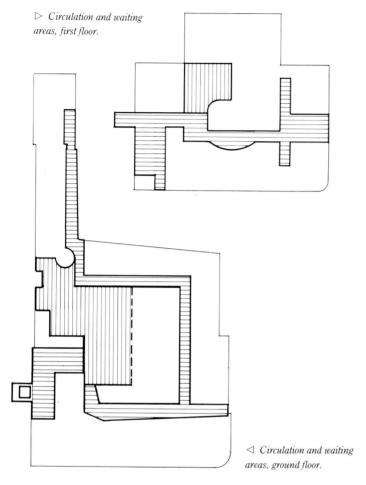

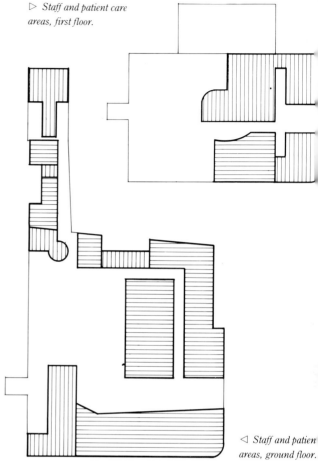

◁ *Circulation and waiting areas, ground floor.*

◁ *Staff and patien areas, ground floor.*

Accessibility to all has been a key feature of the detail design. With barrier-free thresholds, automatic main entrance doors and wide lift doors, wheelchair users – whether staff or public – can also use the purpose-designed reception desk in comfort. There is Braille control in the lift, and contrasting colours to floor finishes at level changes. A flexible sign system provides information in English, Chinese, Bengali and there is also a Bengali speaking health aid on the staff.

Waiting area – mental health
Tea bar
WCs including disabled access.

Patient care
Health education area
Clinic rooms (× 6)
Treatment room clinic
Treatment room GP
Interview (× 2)
Mental health interview (× 3)

Main activity areas

Patients
Main entrance
Pram park
Waiting area clinic
Waiting area – GPs
Waiting area – dental

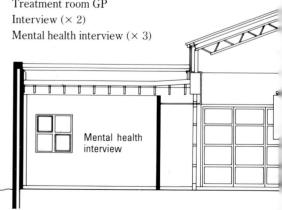

Mental health interview

GP consulting room
GP examination room
Dental education room
Orthodontics
Meeting room

Staff

Main reception
GP reception
Records – clinic
Records – GP
GP common room
Clinic staff common room
X-ray
Laboratory dark room
District nurse office
Administration office
Staff teaching
Staff WC

Comment

The Crowndale Centre is an example of a genuine community public space in both aesthetic and functional terms. It is a result of the London Borough of Camden's five year attempt to create a multi-use building which provides a selection of public and private services which support and respond to the local community under one roof.

Stylistically the interior of the Crowndale main building comes as an exciting surprise, particularly as the old facia of the original building – the post office – hides a striking, user-friendly contemporary interior.

Its focal heart is the glorious four-storey atrium, the scale of which is further dramatized by the low-level ceiling in the lobby/information area.

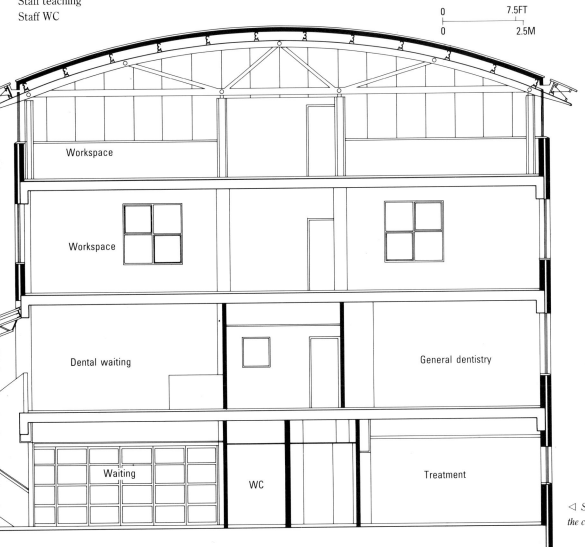

◁ *Section through A–A of the centre.*

▷ The centre looking due west from the car park with the main Crowndale Centre in the background. Photography: Jo Reid and John Peck.

▽ The Crowndale Centre looking south. The new roof to the main building offers just a clue to the dramatic transformation inside. The main entrance is in Eversholt Street on the right, from which the health centre is also accessed. On the horizon is St Paul's Cathedral. Photography: Jo Reid and John Peck.

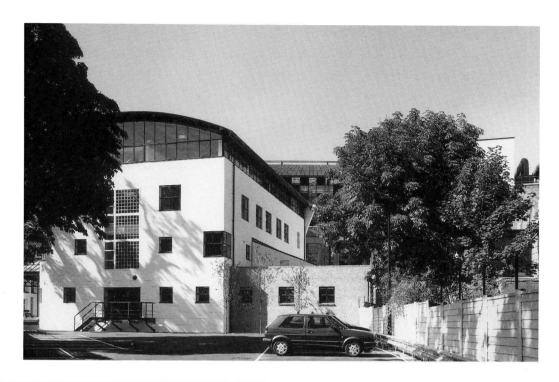

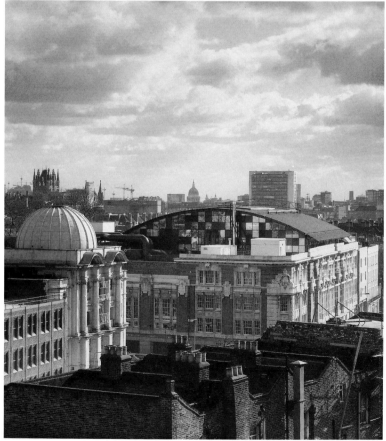

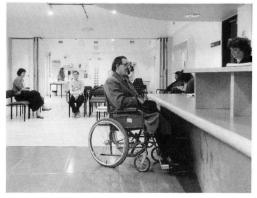

△ The main reception desk is sensitively designed to accommodate wheelchair visitors/users. Photography: Peter Cook.

As with the main building, the health centre's heart is a light glazed area with a slanted roof which forms a conservatory-like reception area. There is a strong simple modernist structural form with an emphasis on natural materials and abundant glazing.

Notwithstanding its architectural merits, the Crowndale Centre's very existence is an achievement. It is a triumph of community enterprise. Such innovation was based upon Rock

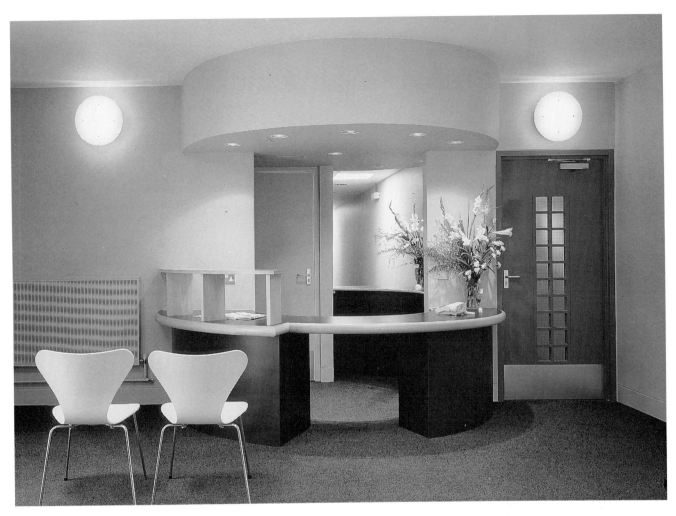

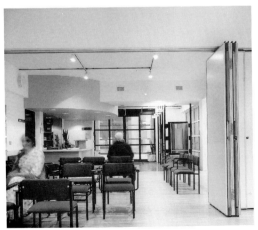

△ *Looking back towards the health centre entrance and reception. In the foreground the folding doors can be* utilized to sub-divide the space for use in health education programmes. *Photography: Peter Cook.*

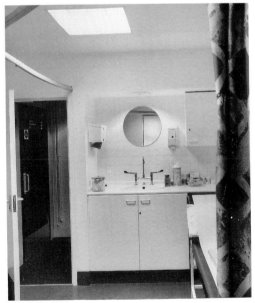

△ *The sub-reception desk for the GP surgery taken from the GP waiting area with access to the consulting rooms via the door on the right. Photography: Jo Reid and John Peck.*

◁ *The GP consulting room. View of wash hand basin and clinical store with the examination couch on the right. In contrast to many GP-led primary health care centres, the doctor's surgery is almost on the periphery of the health centre rather than its focal point. Photography: Peter Cook.*

Townsend's experience of generating possibilities for mixed-use facilities elsewhere in London.

The significance of the health centre as part of this development focuses primary care as a truly community resource.

As Wendy Mason, the project architect, states:

On the same site a visitor can obtain health care, advice from their social worker and a cup of tea in generous, bright and modern surroundings. Previously there has been a tendency for public buildings to be designed for omnipotent unresponsive and remote bureaucracies. The Crowndale Centre is a building for the community.

Despite the integration of social, community and health services, the GP's surgery remains almost autonomous. This is possibly due to different forms of funding in relation to health authority expenditure and the independent nature of the general practitioner. However, as the health centre evolves the surgery element will no doubt become more integrated as part of the centre.

The opportunities for a fully integrated primary health care facility have been created by a forward-looking client together with an architect who has assumed a great role as 'enabler' to make such an important and much needed project happen.

Mixed use developments such as the Crowndale can offer both health and commercial sectors real benefit. The commercial sector benefits by having a natural and reliable source of attracting visitors on site who then can make use of the developer's other facilities and services. The health care sector benefits primarily from the reduced cost of not having to develop a stand-alone facility. It also enables the health centre to function as a drop-in facility. This allows greater opportunities for success in preventive and health education programmes. With a more informal means of access, the visitor can make use of a number of services within the centre obviating the need for a special journey to the clinic.

The Andover Medical Centre

Location:	**Islington, North London**
Completed:	**June 1987**
Type of facility:	**Group practice premises for four doctors**
Architect:	**Cassidy Taggart Partnership**
Client:	**Drs Shenfield, Amin, Chaudhri and Haikel**
Gross floor area:	**296 sq m (3185 sq ft)**
Photography:	**Dennis Gilbert**

Architect's statement:
Tom Reynolds, Project Architect Associate, Cassidy Taggart Partnership

Our client, a four doctor practice, with a list of 10,000 patients in Islington, North London, approached us in June 1984 to assist them in building a new medical centre to replace two run down and cramped premises they were currently working in. Several years prior to our appointment the doctors had enlisted the help of the Polytechnic of North London's Medical Architecture Research Unit to help them in their search for a site.

The site eventually selected and acquired from Islington Borough Council was a grassed, open space measuring 30 × 24 m (98 ft 5 in × 78 ft 9 in) on the Hornsey Road, a busy and noisy thoroughfare lined by an incohesive mixture of council, residential, commercial and social buildings. It is overlooked from the rear by a large housing estate and lies between a police station to the north and Newington Borough Way (a feeder road to the housing estate) and a fire station to the south.

The primary environmental criteria dictated by this site were as follows:

- Maintain maximum outlet from the adjacent houses on the estate that previously enjoyed uninterrupted views over the open space.
- Protect the building and remaining open space from the noise and traffic pollution of Hornsey Road.

- Provide a secure protective facade to Hornsey Road and Newington Borough Way.
- Provide a gateway to the estate.

The doctors' prime concern was that the proposed new premises should be as open and light as possible, providing a pleasant and efficient place to work in and for patients to visit.

Their requirements for light and openness and efficiency, combined with these environmental factors, resulted in the concept of a walled garden from which the building could be entered and which could also be viewed from both the waiting space of the medical centre as well as the adjacent houses on the estate. Access for the disabled and elderly dictated that the majority of the accommodation should be on the ground floor which in turn led to the building being single storey. The L-shaped wall extends the full length of both Newington Borough Way and Hornsey Road, and is made up of cellular spaces – the consulting rooms, nursing room, treatment room, conference room, office and toilets. Nestled between these walls is the waiting space providing an embryonic and restful environment for the patients. The problem of a cold, north facing waiting space was countered by raising the roof over this area to provide a triangular clerestory to capture maximum sunlight penetrating from the south.

The reception area is placed at the fulcrum of the triangle providing easy access from all points of the building and allowing full visual links to public areas.

Half-screened circulation spaces between the consulting rooms and the waiting area provide a degree of privacy when the consulting room doors are open, and also provide a protective means of discreet exits for distressed patients.

The immediate accessibility between the waiting room and the consulting rooms is designed to allow patients to wait adjacent to their respective consulting room. As such, this avoids the design stereotype of long and often wasteful circulation spaces.

The staff are provided with a private entrance which leads through the staff conference room to

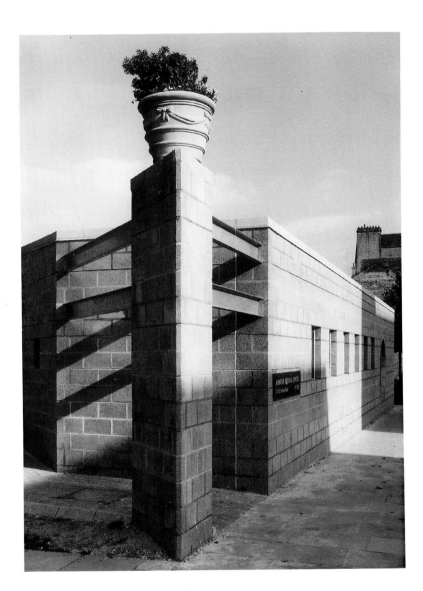

the heart of the building. The consulting rooms, treatment rooms and nursing rooms are provided with a 400 mm sq (1 ft 4 inch square) window facing south or south-west. These are double-glazed and fitted with acoustic ventilators to allow ventilation while keeping noise penetration to a minimum. The office enjoys a circular window allowing light penetration while retaining the majority of external wall space to be taken up by records storage.

△ *The Andover Medical Centre, Hornsey Road, Islington, London.*

▷ *The site was originally a neglected open space on the busy and noisy Hornsey Road. It is located opposite a petrol station. The centre's neighbours are a police and fire station. An uncompromising urban location.*

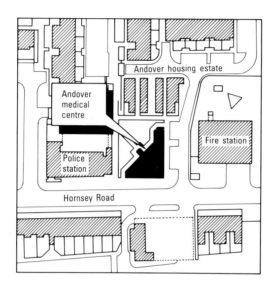

Andover housing estate

Andover medical centre

Fire station

Police station

Hornsey Road

Construction

Mass concrete strip foundations with block cavity walls filled with lean mix concrete. Reinforced concrete floor slab on hard core. Insulation below floor screed. External walls are cavity insulated block work walls Fir faced inside and out. Internal walls are Fir faced concrete block. The flat roof over the cellar rooms is comprised of timber joists, furrings, insulation plywood deck and asphalt. The pitch roof over the waiting room is constructed on a steel structural frame with timber joists, insulated and covered in galvanized steel sheet colour-coated. Ceilings are painted plaster board. There is aluminium double-glazed curtain walling to the waiting room with aluminium double-glazing windows to doors elsewhere.

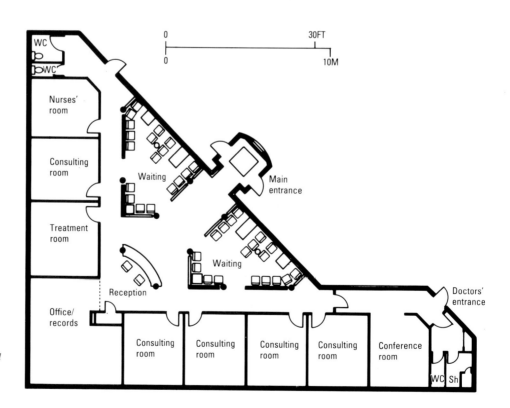

▷ *Ground-floor plan. Within the sanctuary of a walled garden courtyard, the centre has a symmetrical plan with the reception desk acting as its focal point.*

Main activity areas

Public
Main entrance
Waiting area (× 2)
WCs

Patient care
Treatment room
Visitors' consulting room
GP's consulting room (× 4)

Staff
Nurse's office
Reception
Office/records
Staff room
WCs and shower
Staff entrance

Comment

As standalone buildings, practice premises such as the Andover Medical Centre can often do little to make an effective impact on such hostile inner city environments. The architectural language of 'reflecting the local scale of an area' or 'within keeping of the locality' is quite simply not understood on the streets.

The architects were in a sense reacting against the dynamics of the site and therefore created a defensive wall to fend off the elements of the outside world and create a haven of order and balance inside.

As illustrated at Manor Place (page 113) whilst the site does present a difficult set of constraints,

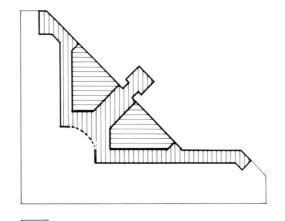

◁ *Circulation and waiting areas.*

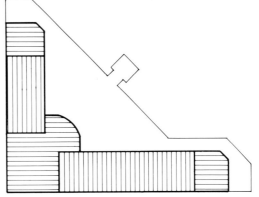

◁ *Patient care and staff.*

▽ *Section through the centre showing the clerestory window offering natural light into the waiting and reception areas.*

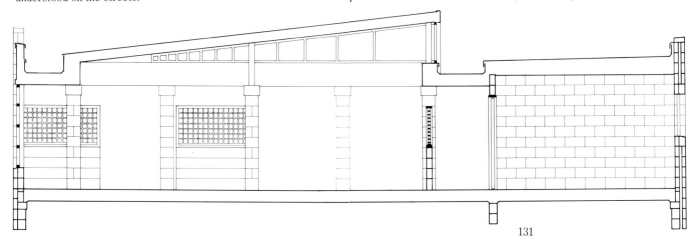

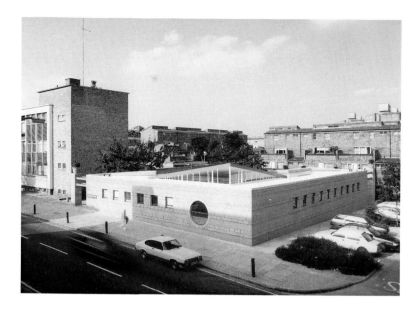

◁ The centre viewed from the south-west. The building responds to the site by using the internal wall as a shield to protect the activities inside from its urban location.

the identification and purchase of suitable sites for primary care in inner cities is becoming an increasingly difficult task. Within such densely populated and built environments the competition for quality sites often pushes their price out of the reach of health providers. Even once a site has been identified, town planning (zoning authorities) need to be convinced that a primary health care facility will not aggravate already existing problems of traffic and car parking.

In terms of its geographical location, the centre is however easily accessible for its patients.

▽ The inner courtyard. As the visitor approaches the entrance lobby there is a subtle glimpse into the centre through the circular window. Visitors are unobtrusively observed by the receptionist. From the waiting area patients in turn can observe the comings and goings of the courtyard and also supervise any parked prams or cycles.

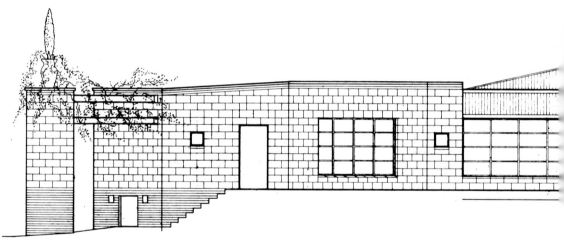

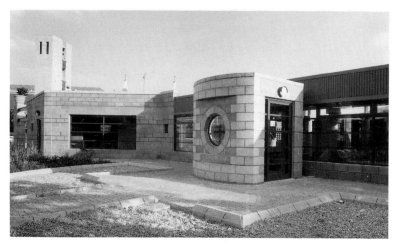

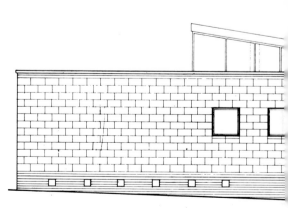

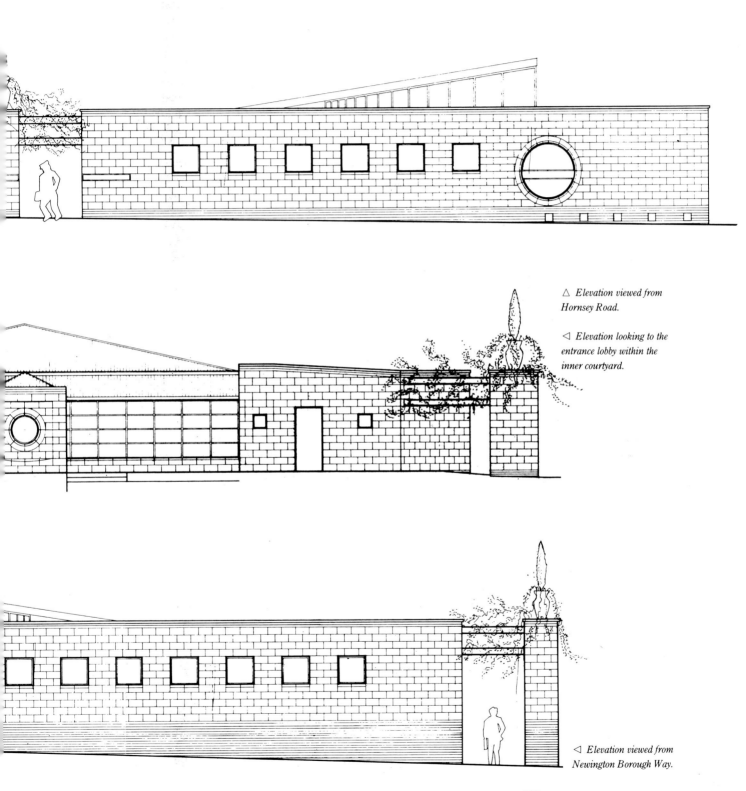

△ Elevation viewed from
Hornsey Road.

◁ Elevation looking to the
entrance lobby within the
inner courtyard.

◁ Elevation viewed from
Newington Borough Way.

133

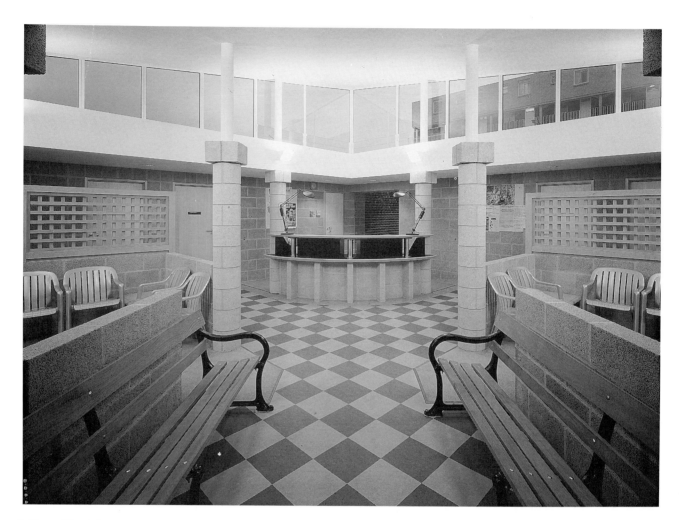

△ *The reception desk as viewed from the main entrance lobby. The waiting areas are on either side. The timber screens offer visual privacy to the consulting room doors. Note the bench seats were temporarily positioned inside the centre pending completion of the external landscape.*

▷ *Perspective illustrating route from entry to courtyard from Hornsey Road.*

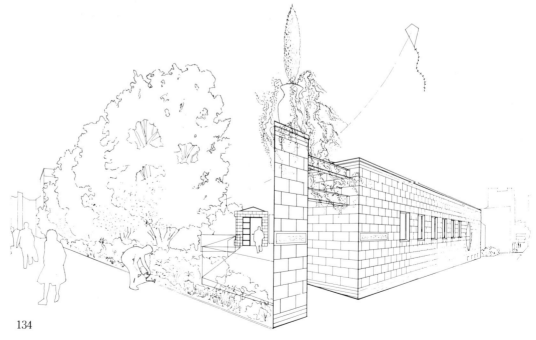

134

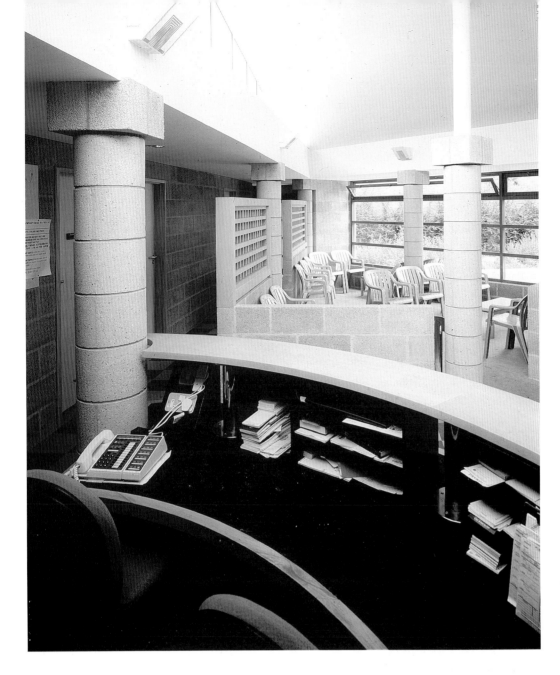

◁ View from reception
desk on to one of the two
waiting areas which in turn
looks on to the walled
courtyard. Note how the
waiting chairs face away
from the corridor serving the
clinical rooms on the left.
This, together with the
screen, allows for visual
privacy to and from these
rooms.

Upon entering the walled courtyard garden the symmetry, simplicity and logic of the whole arrangement is of immediate benefit, particularly to the first-time visitor.

The main entrance stands out from the building profile and if approached from either the east or west (which most would) the footpath guides the visitor directly to the main doors. Once inside the lobby the reception can be located, not only by its central location but also by the flood of daylight that bathes the desk from the clerestory lights above.

From reception, patients are directed to one of the two waiting areas. The split waiting layout breaks down the scale of the space and allows for a shorter, more direct route from waiting to consultation.

Visual privacy is maintained by the use of a screened wall between the waiting area and the circulation area to the clinical rooms. This factor is further enhanced by the arrangement of the waiting chairs which face back on to the courtyard. This therefore acts as a focal point and a useful distraction from the comings and goings of the clinical rooms. This arrangement of fragmenting the waiting space and direct access to the consulting rooms (i.e. the corridor-less surgery) echoes the concept of the Store Heddinge Health Centre, Denmark (page 149). In a quieter site location, audio privacy could have been a problem with only one door and a relatively short distance separating the conversations within the consulting rooms and the waiting room. However, such is the intensity of

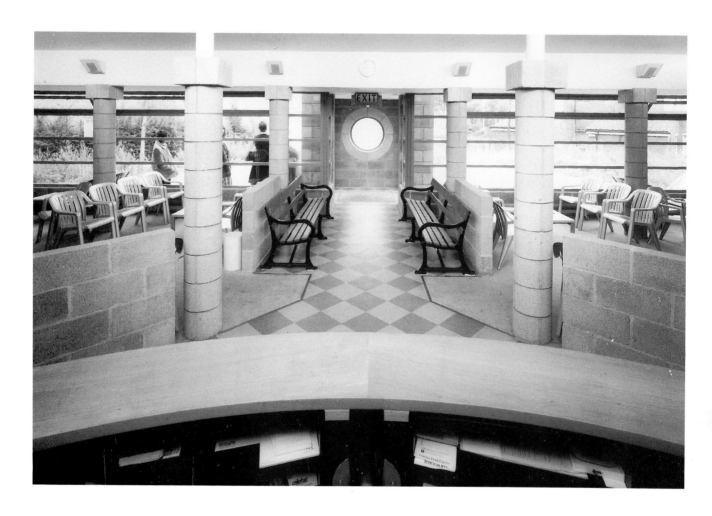

△ *Security is 'designed in' to the building by ensuring that all those who enter and leave the building are supervised from the reception point.*

background noise that this tends to mask normal levels of conversation. Indeed the background level of noise is so high that the problem has been one of containing transmission of sound from the Hornsey Road into the consulting rooms, rather than sound from the consulting rooms to the waiting areas.

Each of the clinical rooms, and even the staff room, is of approximately the same size. This has allowed for flexibility of use even during its comparatively brief history. The staff entrance by the consulting suite also allows for the distressed patient to discreetly leave the centre without having to walk past the main entrance.

The simplicity of the design solution at the

Andover Medical Centre is the result of a sophisticated approach to a complex set of criteria in terms of the site as previously discussed, whilst satisfying the medical planning requirements. Great attention has been paid to the interior design and details which offer an environment which borrows little from either a clinical or domestic interior.

Since its completion the exterior walls have been daubed with graffiti. However, the centre's tough outer shell remains protective of its inner sanctuary. Perhaps the graffiti can be viewed as a symbol of the building's acceptance and initiation within an uncompromising urban environment as the 'new kid on the block'.

Finland

Population 1990:	**4.97 million**
Percentage of population aged 65 plus:	**13**
Population estimated year 2020:	**5.04 million**
Percentage of population aged 65 plus (2020):	**19.9**
Health care expenditure in pounds per person:	**732**
Health care expenditure expressed as percentage of GNP:	**6.7**

(Source: Compendium of Health Statistics, Office of Health Economics, London, UK.)

When Finland became independent in 1917 a period of vigorous development began. Economic growth also enabled the development of health care. Medical science as well as training of health care personnel made rapid progress.

At the beginning of the century tuberculosis had become a serious national disease which was fought on many frontiers. At the end of the 1920s 18 tuberculosis sanitoria had been built in the country. These included acclaimed examples by the architects Alvar Aalto and Jussi Paatela.

An improvement in the status of mental care was also considered to be important. Within a short period of time 14 new district mental hospitals were built in addition to the three existing ones. The hospitals were owned by communal federations but received considerable state subsidies. This was therefore a response to the treatment of special conditions, especially tuberculosis, through the provision of purpose-built facilities. However, as tuberculosis became more preventable through immunization programmes, such buildings were largely redundant. Today Finland is evaluating how best to re-use these institutions which, generally, are located far away from main population centres.

Health care in the community

The network of community-based hospitals expanded rapidly. At the beginning of the 1950s there were more than 100 community hospitals. Posts of communal physicians were not, however, established at the rate the government expected. At the beginning of the 1950s a directive was given stipulating that in communes with more than 8000 inhabitants and in towns with more than 30,000 it was necessary to establish two posts of communal or municipal physicians. A more notable improvement in this respect was achieved only in the 1970s when the Primary Health Care Act (1972) was passed.

Maternal and child health care (MCH) services were started in the period between the world wars, but the real growth came only in the 1940s. In 1940 there were 300 MCH centres; by the 1950s there were more than 6000.

Today health care is split into two levels: primary health care and specialized medical treatment. Communes and communal federations maintain both services which are subsidized by the state. The commune, or the communal federation, is responsible for the primary health care and additional treatment of every inhabitant in the commune. Regional and local hospitals are responsible for specialized medical treatment. The system is hierarchic. Since the Primary Health.Care Act of 1972 the system and hierarchy have become noticeably clearer and more defined.

The Act respects the principle of communal autonomy. The commune organizes the services with the aid of state subsidies. The goal is a system that covers the entire population, provides free treatment, aims for equality and endeavours to supply complete but integrated services. Other objectives include community participation and close interaction between health centres and inhabitants.

Every commune is obliged to set up a health centre, either on its own or jointly with its neighbour. 'Health centre' however does not mean a single building or building complex, but refers to the organization of supplying services. In practice, most health centres are comprised of units that existed before the Primary Health Care Act took effect, i.e. MCH centres, local doctors' reception points, laboratories, local hospitals and wards, supplemented by new buildings where required.

The minimum population base for a health centre service is 10,000; the only exceptions are smaller bases in certain sparsely inhabited areas to avoid excessive distances. Many communes have therefore been obliged to form federations running joint health centres. Finland currently has just over 200 centres, of which 100 cover single communes and the rest two or more communes.

Health centre services are administered by communal or federation health boards which appoint the staff, draw up and supervise the local plans, and provide a channel for citizen participation so that inhabitants can make their wishes known.

Most health centres have at least four doctors, the absolute minimum is three, to ensure that one doctor is always on duty. Other personnel number roughly 11 per doctor. The centre runs a small laboratory and X-ray department. Nearly all centres include local hospitals with beds, many for observation, mild illness and chronic patients.

The services are supplied in several units, often scattered around the area. Some of them are open day and night, others are visited by health personnel once or twice a week. Except in sparsely populated areas there is usually an MCH centre within pram distance of every mother.

Finland's low infant mortality is largely due to its MCH programmes. Health education also plays an important role, especially for specific target groups. Currently the accent is on health counselling for the old and on family planning. Health education is also given at regular check-ups and screening.

Health centres are responsible for school and student health. They are also obliged to arrange occupational health services where required, but larger employers and companies usually take care of this for their own employees.

Services offered in health centres include physiotherapy, mental health work and other

conditions that can be treated outside the hospital under the care and supervision of a general practitioner. Very few centres have specialist doctors, but these can be consulted when necessary.

Doctors seldom visit patients at home in Finland, but public health nurses often call on elderly patients and others in need of help.

One of the aims of Finnish primary health care is that as many services as possible should be given by public health nurses, midwives, physiotherapists, etc. working in teams.

Private medicine
Public health care in Finland is supplemented by private services, of which private practice specialists in large towns, dental care for adults, physiotherapy, rehabilitation and occupational health care are especially important. With the exception of dental health care for adults, patients receive compensation from sickness insurance.

Under the Primary Health Care Act resources for primary health care were allocated particularly to the country's peripheral regions where the need was greatest. Consequently, development was slower in the cities where private practice still plays a major role in primary health care today. Private practitioners play an even more important role in specialist medicine.

The requirements of physiotherapy and rehabilitation greatly exceed the health centres' resources, so here too the ratio of private practice is high. In some cases, health centres hire services in the private sector.

Reference

Seliger, M. (1986) 'Health for all in Finland', Laakintohallitus Valtion Painatuskeskus.

The Masku Neurological Rehabilitation Centre

Location:	**Masku**
Completed:	**1988**
Type of facility:	**52 patient and visitor centre for the treatment of multiple sclerosis**
Architects:	**Laiho Pulkkinen Raunio**
Client:	**League of Finnish Multiple Sclerosis Associations**
Gross floor area:	**4440 sq m (47,780 sq ft)**
Photography:	**Ola Lalho**

Architect's statement:
Ilpo Raunio

As with the Renfrew Center (page 68) the Masku Neurological Rehabilitation Centre is the first of its kind in Finland. It forms the second of the case study examples which deliberately cross the boundaries defining a community-based primary health care facility. It is therefore interesting to note that today in Finland the term 'health centre' is related more to a service-led rather than building-led health care provision. It can cover, for example, health care in a variety of buildings from outpost MCH centres to local hospitals and wards. It is within this wider context of community health care facilities that the Masku Centre is discussed in terms of its functional and architectural innovations.

Masku Neurological Rehabilitation Centre was commissioned by the League of Finnish Multiple Sclerosis Associations, a private national organization. Within the national organization programming has been going on for the facility since the early 1980s. Actual building design took place from 1985 to 1987, and construction began in 1986. The facility was inaugurated in the early part of 1988. The centre was financed mainly by 'Raha-Automaattiyhdistys', a Finnish organization for legalized gambling which under state supervision has a monopoly in running the slot-machine industry

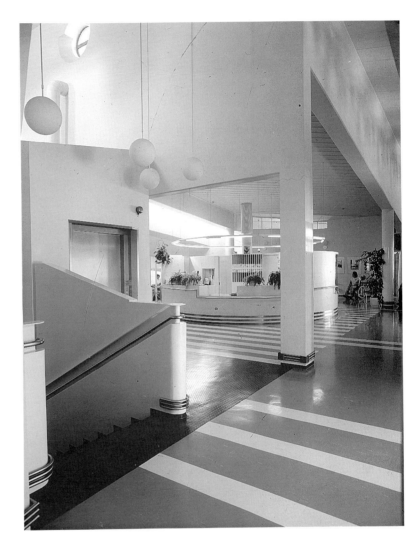

△ *Masku Neurological Rehabilitation Centre, Masku.*

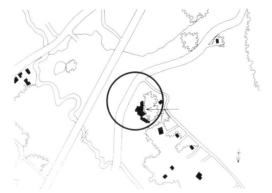

◁ *Location plan. The Centre enjoys a rural setting near the village of Masku which is approximately 20 km (12.5 miles) from Turku.*

139

in Finland. In addition, the League of Finnish Multiple Sclerosis Associations assisted in the financing.

Masku Neurological Rehabilitation Centre is the first facility of its kind in Finland specializing in the care and rehabilitation of MS patients. The centre also provides training facilities for education of personnel in the social service and health fields. There is a total of 52 patient and visitor beds in the facility in single and double rooms, some of them accessible by wheelchair.

A comprehensive rehabilitation plan is constructed for each MS patient by a team which includes a neurologist, a nurse, a physical therapist and a social worker. The therapeutical goal during a period of three weeks is to give the patients renewed means in their struggle for an independent life.

Both the origin and the cure for MS are still unknown. By continuous follow-up and treatment

patients' daily lives can be eased, but the nature of the illness is such that a progressively more restricted and difficult life can be expected. The client's aim was to ease and offer support to the lives of these patients. The architect's brief was simply to create an environment that would be sensitive and cohesive to these aims.

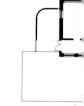

▷ *First-floor plan.*

▷ *Ground-floor plan.*
Because of the levels of the site the main entrance appears at first floor level.

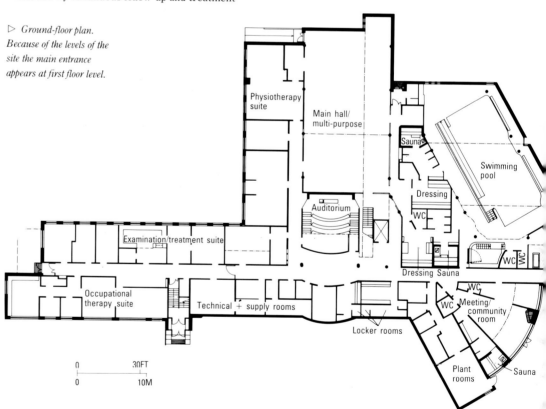

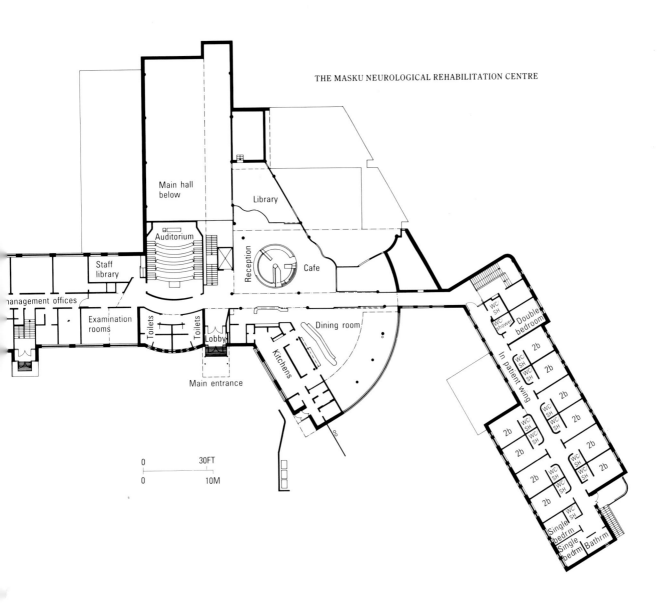

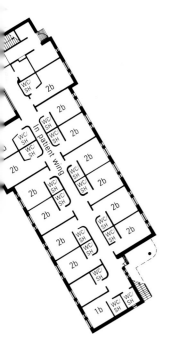

Programming

The main aim of the facility programme was to create sufficient space for the treatment and rehabilitation of all types of neurological illnesses, particularly multiple sclerosis. In addition, spaces were needed for training of care personnel. No prior example existed for the planners and designers to learn from, as facilities of this type are unique.

To the designers the spatial brief appeared as a kind of 'spa hotel' which also included the more normal health centre spaces for reception, examination and treatment. The most challenging factor was that all these spaces had to be designed for people whose daily lives and physical and mental abilities were increasingly affected by MS or other neurological illnesses.

141

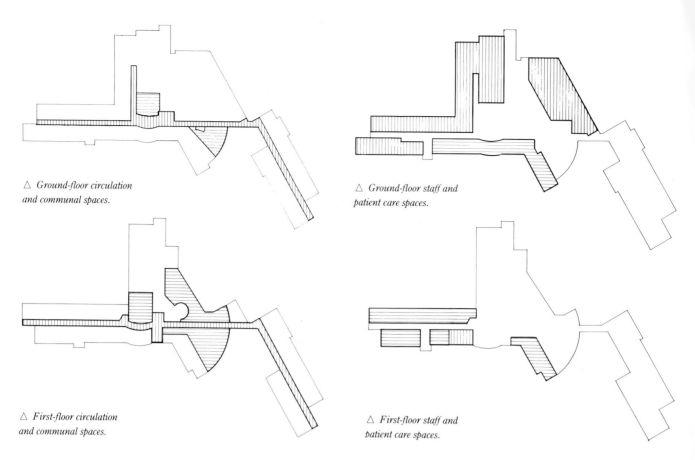

△ *Ground-floor circulation and communal spaces.*

△ *Ground-floor staff and patient care spaces.*

△ *First-floor circulation and communal spaces.*

△ *First-floor staff and patient care spaces.*

Building description

The centre is located 20 km (12.5 miles) west of Turku, Finland, near the village of Masku. The building looks on to rolling, cultivated fields dotted with forested knolls, a landform typical of this part of the country. Farm dwellings are frequently situated where forest meets field. Architecture for

the MS centre has been influenced by this setting and its building form.

The various functions in the building have been arranged around a central hall so that one can glimpse the functions and gain an understanding of the whole immediately upon entering. Common social spaces – a cafe, dining room and library – can all be entered from the central hall. A

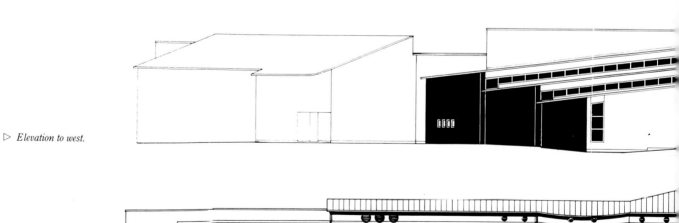

▷ *Elevation to west.*

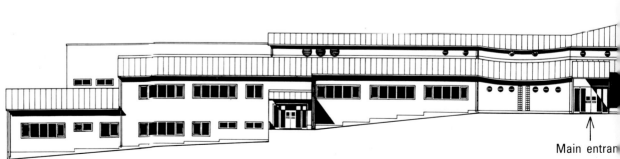

Main entran

142

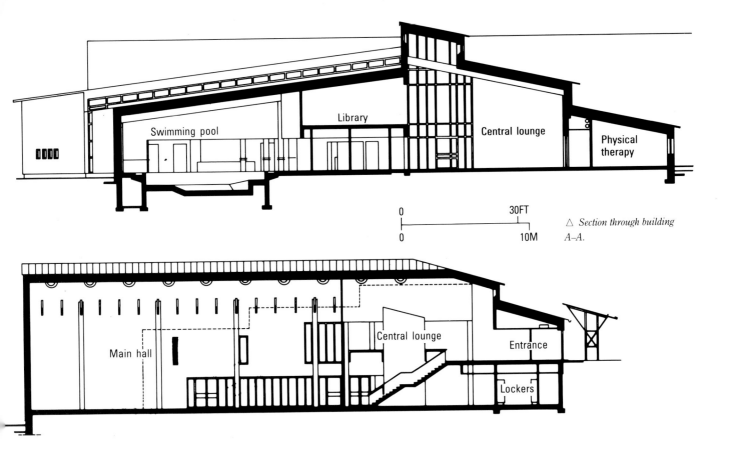

Swimming pool

Library

Central lounge

Physical therapy

0 —————————— 30FT

0 —————————— 10M

△ *Section through building A–A.*

Main hall

Central lounge

Entrance

Lockers

△ *Section through building B–B.*

swimming pool and a large hall for exercise and gatherings can be viewed through windows from the central hall as well. There is a small, terraced auditorium adjacent to the central hall, separate wings for offices and examination rooms and for patients' quarters. The centre offers an abundance of many types of water treatments such as warm water exercise and sauna bathing. These are

typical forms of therapy for the MS patient. Most of these services are located in the lower levels between the exercise hall and the pool. A lift serves the two levels, although both can be entered on ground level as the building is sited on a slope.

All visitors take part in group physiotherapy. The cognitive, psychological and social problems are confronted in group discussions under the control of

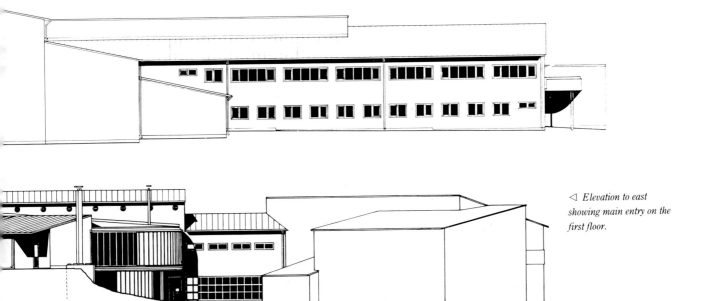

◁ *Elevation to east showing main entry on the first floor.*

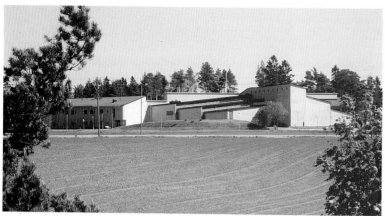

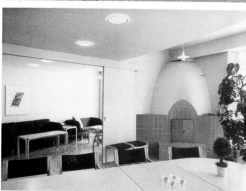

△ *Facade to the north-west towards the village of Masku.*

▷ *The central hall used for exercises amongst other uses performs a major function within the Centre.*

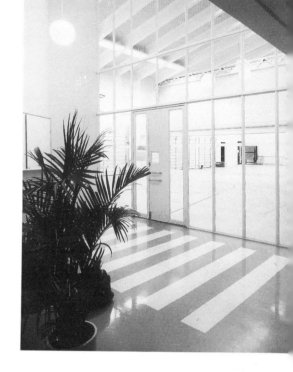

△ *Meeting and community rooms with the fireplace forming a focal point. Attention to interior furniture and details is evident throughout the building.*

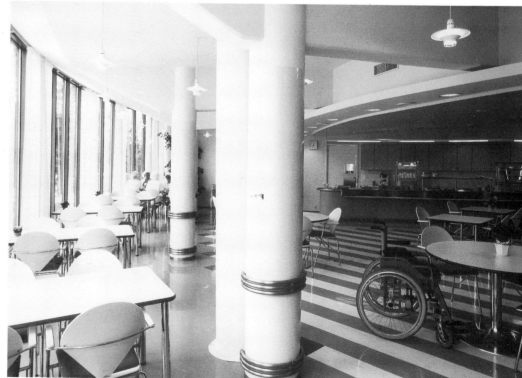

▷ *The dining room looking towards the servery and kitchens. The dining room tables are suitable for wheelchairs as indicated on the right-hand side of this illustration.*

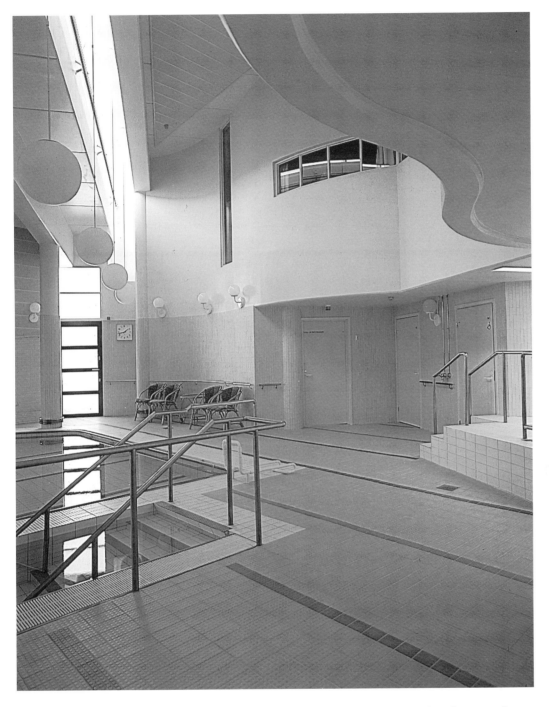

◁ *The swimming pool. The architects have paid great attention to the quality of the spaces in terms of their dual function of therapy and recreation. The style of the interior has a passing reference to the Finnish architect Alvar Aalto.*

a neuropsychologist or social worker. The occupational therapist takes care of the adaptive equipment and wheelchair evaluation. Some of the visitors are taught how to use personal computers as part of the activities of daily life.

The building structure is of concrete. Exterior cladding is of a light tan brick with a similar colour mortar. The overall effect is that of a stuccoed surface. The roof is of sheet metal painted black. Interior colours and materials are generally light and have been selected to help orientation within the building. Only materials that are allergy-tested, easy to clean and do not collect dirt or dust have been utilized.

Main activity areas

Patient treatment rooms
Physical therapy/dressing
Water treatment and massage
Occupational therapy
Examination rooms

Communal spaces
Main hall/multi-purpose
Sauna/dressing
Swimming pool
Meeting/community room
Patio
Central lounge/cafe
Dining room
Library/Auditorium

Patients' rooms
Single bedrooms ($\times$ 4)
Double bedrooms ($\times$ 24)

Staff
Technical and library supply rooms
Locker rooms
Staff library
Administration rooms
Reception
Kitchens

Comment

While the need to provide clinics for the treatment of tuberculosis has all but disappeared, facilities such as the Masku Centre are sadly much needed for a disease for which, at present, there is no cure.

Unlike facilities such as nursing homes, or even hospices, patients do not come here to live. Instead it provides a base for day care and extended treatment over a three week period. It is therefore a community-based resource rather than a permanent residential facility.

Its patients are 'visitors', interacting with and as part of the community. As with the Renfrew Center the design and project team were working on a project without precedent. It is perhaps because of this that the design solution carries a refreshing clarity in its planned form and the zoning of the various activities. The bedrooms are situated away from the main functional areas, as are the staff offices.

The formality of both these spaces is expressed as simply double-loaded corridor areas, yet in contrast the building begins to loosen and fragment around the communal activity areas. The communal spaces of dining and cafe are located around the hub of the reception area, looking out to both the outside countryside as well as across the swimming pool on the lower ground floor.

The tragedy of multiple sclerosis is its effect on a person's physical and mental capabilities. With the advent of such dual disabilities, sufferers have to come to terms with a changing lifestyle. At best the condition may stabilize, yet all sufferers, together with their families and friends, will suffer frustration as parts of their lives slip away.

The Masku Centre offers a sensitive and, in many ways, an uplifting environment for support and treatment. It welcomes its visitors within an informal and certainly non-institutional setting. The nature of treatment is therapeutic rather than clinical. The building is therefore far removed from that of a hospital. It is also lavish and rich in terms of the spaces it offers to its patients within a relaxed setting. This symbolizes that all that is possible can be done. What a contrast to those depressing day centres for the handicapped, where hard working staff struggle to offer care and support often within totally inadequate and under-funded premises.

As a new type of building, no doubt important lessons will be learned as its users adjust to the new facility. The Renfrew Center, for example, changed the use of some rooms after a period of operation. In Finland, where health centres refer to a network of services rather than a specific building, the Masku Centre has an important role.

146

Denmark

Population 1990:	**5.12 million**
Percentage of population aged 65 plus:	**15.4**
Population estimated year 2020:	**4.80 million**
Percentage of population aged 65 plus (2020):	**21.2**
Health care expenditure in pounds per person:	**777**
Health care expenditure expressed as percentage of GNP:	**6.7**

(Source: Compendium of Health Statistics, Office of Health Economics, London, UK.)

Denmark is recognized as a pioneer in the development of its welfare state and national health service systems. It has set the pattern for its Nordic neighbours of Sweden, Finland, Iceland and Norway.

The national health insurance scheme guarantees the right to free medical treatment by a medical practitioner or practising consultant. This right is independent of a person's income. Costs of the service are paid through rates and taxes by the 14 county hospital authorities and the city councils of Copenhagen and Frederiksberg.

Danish primary health services are centred around general practitioner services. The Danish health care system allows patients to choose their own doctor.

There are many similarities with the United Kingdom system. The general practitioner operates as an independent contractor and undertakes his business independently of hospital services. In practice, however, his income is derived from the service he carries out for the public health insurance. This is calculated according to a scale of fees determined by the doctor's own professional organization and the Public Health Insurance Board.

General practitioners often collaborate with other doctors, either in partnership or group practices. They tend to own their own practice premises and are also responsible for the employment and salaries of assistants such as secretaries, nurses, etc.

The setting up of a new practice is controlled and regulated according to an agreement with the public health insurance. Each new practice must be approved.

General practitioners are required to hold open consultation sessions four times per week in the mornings and once a week late in the afternoons. GPs are under obligation to give consultations to all those patients who report during surgery hours, and further without any extra remuneration they must undertake home visits so long as they are notified between the hours of 8.00 and 9.00 in the morning.

On average, between 30 and 40 patients attend the private practitioner every day and he may visit three to four patients at home. The visits and consultations cover anything from the more complicated clinical examinations to new ailments to renewal of prescriptions and other minor tasks.

In the majority of cases, general practitioners will be able to undertake the necessary examination and treatment themselves with the facilities available to them in their consulting rooms. A small proportion of patients will be referred for further examination and treatment to either practising specialists or hospitals.

The general practitioner has a considerable degree of contact with the municipal or county social welfare services. It is often the GP, in his capacity as family doctor, who is aware of social problems which the family may be unable to resolve without the help of the Department of Social Affairs. Further, GPs are responsible for issuing medical certificates in connection with sickness benefits and the provision of visiting nursing services, etc. Similarly they play an important role with respect to recommending patients for nursing homes and applying on the patient's behalf for disability or other pensions.

An increasingly important part of primary health care is the concern with health education and maternity care. Expectant mothers have the right to free medical examinations before giving birth and two after. Advice is also given on family planning. Examinations are carried out by general practitioners but in close collaboration with the hospital services departments for obstetrics. There is a further provision for at least five examinations by a midwife.

The national health service has set up directives for maternity care services to ensure that women in all parts of the country are provided with facilities of comparable standards.

Child health care

Health service authorities are notified of births by the midwife in the municipality where the mother lives. They in turn offer health care facilities to the mother in the form of home visits by a health worker.

On average each child is visited on between seven and nine occasions during its first year, but this can vary considerably depending upon the needs of the individual child or family. The aim of the health worker (health visitor) is to give basic and individual health guidance to the parents to arrange for the family doctor or social welfare expertise as and when required.

Health workers, in co-operation with medical and social welfare workers, aim to prevent the occurrence of illness and to recognize potential development and growing problems in children at the earliest possible stage.

Child examinations

All children can take advantage of a programme which provides ten health examinations before reaching school age and vaccinations against whooping cough (Pertusis), diphtheria, tetanus and poliomyelitis.

These examinations and vaccinations are carried out by the private practitioners, often in close collaboration with the health worker. The great majority of families in Denmark take advantage of these facilities.

Occupational health services

Legislation has been passed to give all industrial

concerns the opportunity to establish occupational health services. In factories with special safety problems these services are mandatory. Occupational health services are still in the development stage, but it is intended that they will encompass medical, economical and technical expertise, which will be offered in close collaboration with the concern's industrial safety organizations.

Occupational health services get support in the form of advice and supervision, partly from the Industrial Inspection Services and partly from the industrial medical clinics and out-patients departments which are gradually being established within hospitals in all of the hospital authorities.

Practising specialists

The primary health care service also includes practising specialists who are connected to the national health insurance scheme.

The largest group working within primary health care services are the ear, nose and throat specialists and ophthalmists. These disciplines have entered into special agreements with the National Health Insurance Scheme which, in the case of Copenhagen and Frederiksberg City Councils, differ from the rest of the country. A large proportion of the total out-patient activity for ENT and ophthalmy is undertaken by practising specialists.

A large number of other disciplines also have agreements with the National Health Insurance Scheme. General practitioners can refer their patients for examination and, if necessary, treatment to practising specialists in psychiatry, internal medicine, surgery, gynaecology, obstetrics, dermatology, physiology, etc. In Copenhagen and Frederiksberg a large number of private clinics exist for diagnostic radiology, whilst the out-patient facilities for this discipline throughout the rest of the country are found in hospitals.

At present the Danish health insurance regulations allow patients to choose one of two insurance groups, Group 1 and Group 2. Patients insured in Group 1 are covered for all medical expenses but have to choose one particular private practitioner who they should use in order to get their expenses fully covered. Normally these patients are allowed to change their doctor once a year. They may not go directly to a practising specialist themselves, but must be referred by their own private practitioner. Those patients who choose Group 2 must pay part of the consultation expenses themselves, usually in the order of 25% of the full amount. However, the patient is not obliged to be registered with one particular doctor, and is not dependent on the doctor's referral to attend a practising specialist.

Patients may choose which of the two insurance groups to belong to. Approximately 90% belong to Group 1.

General practitioners in Copenhagen and Frederiksberg are remunerated by the National Health Insurance Scheme annually with a sum which relates to the number of patients registered with them. This is irrespective of the number of times the patient visits the doctor, or by which services the doctor renders the patient.

General practitioners throughout the rest of the country are remunerated by the National Health Insurance Scheme partly according to the numbers of patients on their lists, and partly to the services which they render to the patient. The fees are fixed so that about half is determined by the number of patients, and half by the services provided.

As with other Scandinavian countries the health centre concept has become the focal point for the delivery of primary health care services.

Over the past 25 years many health centres (Laeghuse) have been built. From such centres the GP and other members of the health care team (as described above) offer their primary health care services, which also includes first-aid. In contrast with the United Kingdom, however, GPs in Denmark are not subsidized by the health service for the provision of practice premises.

The Medical Centre, Store Heddinge

Location:	**Store Heddinge, Stevns**
Completed:	**1971**
Type of facility:	**General practitioner practice premises for six doctors plus support staff**
Architects:	**Karsten Vibild MAA (with Finn Sønderbaek & Bent Falk).**
Client:	**Stevns General Practitioners Company, Stevnslaegernes Ejd A/S, Store Heddinge**
Gross floor area:	**520 sq m (5600 sq ft) plus basement area of 90 sq m (970 sq ft). Total: 610 sq m (6600 sq ft)**
Photography:	**Reersø/Karsten Vibild**

Architect's statement:

Co-operation between General Practitioners in specially designed premises offers numerous benefits in the form of group practices in which the doctor assumes joint responsibility for:

- Patient care
- Secretarial services
- Laboratory
- First-aid post
- Finances

As a result of extensive preparatory work, the GPs in the Stevns area were probably the first major group in Denmark to decide upon this highly-integrated form of co-operation. Such co-operation provides the possibility of a much higher efficiency of work. At the same time the shared use and costs of more sophisticated and expensive equipment enables the practitioners to offer the patients better and more comprehensive examination and treatment facilities. A further advantage lies in the introduction of a system of appointments to shorten unnecessary waiting time, while at the same time emergency situations can be dealt with. Likewise,

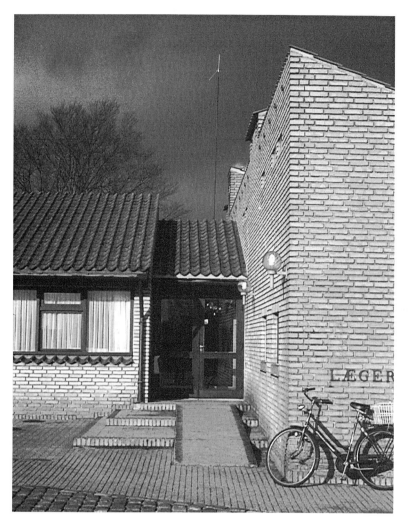

the considerable problem of further education of the doctors can be managed with greater ease.

On this basis the Stevns Doctor Partnership was founded on 1st July 1968. They decided to form a limited property company to be put in charge of the building of the medical centre. The centre was financed by the doctors via a real estate company in which each doctor owned a share. There is no financial support or subsidy from public authorities for doctors' health centres.

Geographically, Stevns is a fairly well defined area and all doctors in the area have joined the group. The medical centre was established in the main town of Store Heddinge, adjacent to the new Town Hall, providing a natural and useful daily working relationship with the social security and welfare office. The practice consists of six doctors. This is considered an appropriate size allowing good opportunities between the members of staff for collaboration in relation to the physical size of the centre.

The practitioners developed their brief with the architects. Particular attention was paid to the need for good internal communication, with a strong emphasis of the ambience on the waiting area. There was also the concern that the building would fit in harmoniously with the scale of the small provincial town around it.

The building takes the form of four clinical blocks of approximately 42 sq m (450 sq ft) with tiled roofs clustered around a timber supported central hall.

△ *Store Heddinge Medical Centre, Store Heddinge.*

▷ *Location plan. The Centre is adjacent to the local Town Hall, both buildings forming the Town Hall square. It is therefore very much a part of the local community.*

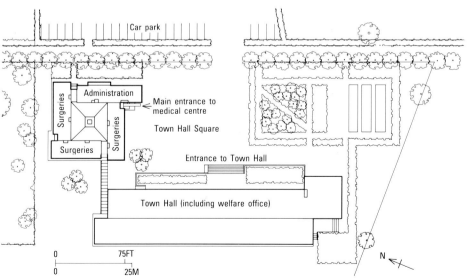

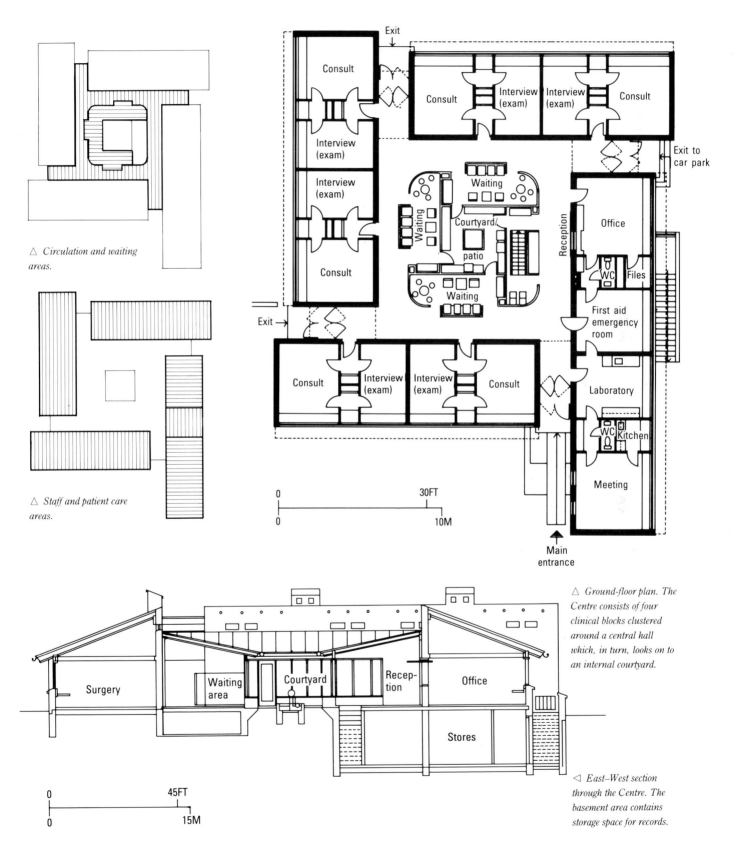

△ *Circulation and waiting areas.*

△ *Staff and patient care areas.*

Exit

Consult

Consult | Interview (exam) | Interview (exam) | Consult

Exit to car park

Interview (exam)

Interview (exam)

Waiting

Waiting

Courtyard/ patio

Reception

Office

WC | Files

First aid emergency room

Laboratory

WC | Kitchen

Consult

Consult | Interview (exam) | Interview (exam) | Consult

Waiting

Exit

Meeting

0   30FT

0   10M

Main entrance

△ *Ground-floor plan. The Centre consists of four clinical blocks clustered around a central hall which, in turn, looks on to an internal courtyard.*

Surgery | Waiting area | Courtyard | Reception | Office

Stores

0   45FT

0   15M

◁ *East–West section through the Centre. The basement area contains storage space for records.*

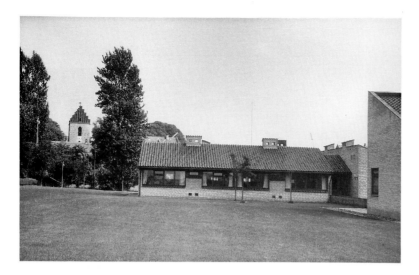

△ West elevation on the right of the gable wall of the town hall. Both buildings are constructed in yellow brick with red roof tiles. The local church can be seen in the background on the left.

each surgery block, and these areas are further sub-divided for children and adults. Corridor space has been minimized. Patients' telephones and toilets have been placed in a small basement section, together with the necessary filing and storage rooms.

In order to avoid sound transmission, each unit has its own separate heating, ventilating and electrical installation. The electrical installation includes an internal communication and signal system.

The building is characterized by traditional building materials, bricks and pine timber, used in their natural texture and colour.

A possible future extension for special functions (chiropody, eye and ear specialists, etc.) has been accommodated to the north side.

Three of the blocks each contain a pair of double surgeries, and the fourth houses shared facilities: secretariat, first-aid room, laboratory and meeting room. Each GP has a double unit consisting of two separate surgeries connected by sound lobbies. The central hall serves as a reception and waiting area, and surrounds a small patio with a fountain and water sculpture. The hall is sub-divided by light screens and low-seating walls into waiting areas for

Main activity areas

Patient
Waiting zone for children
Waiting zone for adults
Public telephones
Patient WCs

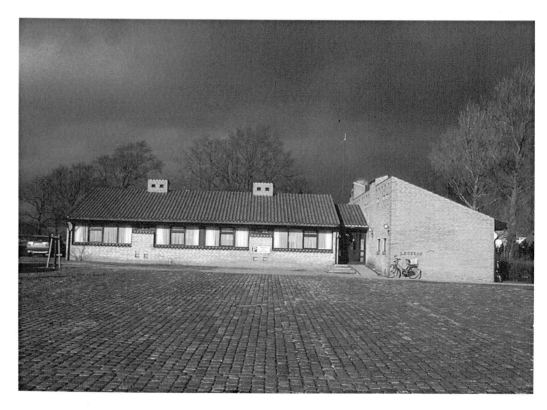

▷ Main entrance from Town Hall square. To cater for the handicapped visitor the stairs are flanked by a ramp.

152

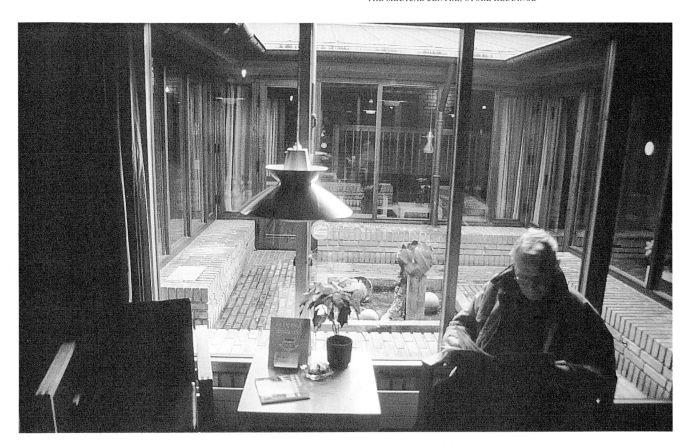

Patient care
First-aid (treatment)
Consulting rooms (× 6)
Interview/examination (× 6)

Staff
Reception
Stores
Office and records store
Laboratory
Pantry/tea kitchen
Meeting room
Staff
WCs

Comment

Although built in the 1970s the Store Heddinge
Medical Centre has been included because it has
important lessons for the 1990s in terms of its
simplicity and wider application.

Despite the complex design requirements for

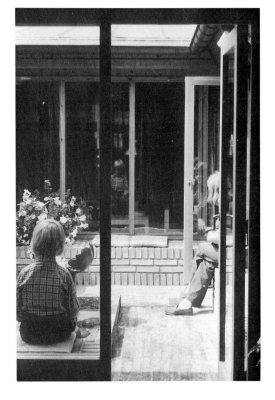

△ *The waiting zone looks
on to an internal courtyard
with a bronze water
sculpture as a focal point,
created by Jens-Flemming
Sorensen. Note the attention
to interior fittings as found
in many Scandinavian
projects.*

◁ *The courtyard, which
also provides brick benches,
can be accessed during
summer months and
enjoyed as part of the
waiting space.*

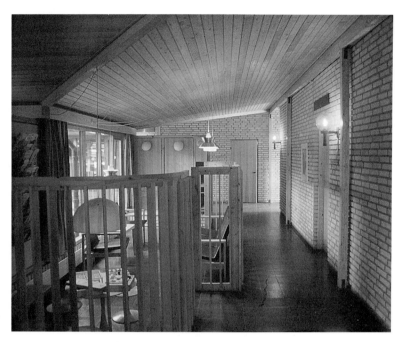

△ The waiting area is divided by partial-height screens into smaller sub-waiting zones around the central patio; each however, is within sight and a short walking distance of the consulting rooms. Confidentiality is achieved by utilizing double door access via a sound lobby off the main circulation area.

primary health care facilities this centre manages to offer a simple, yet sophisticated, solution. Standing alongside the Town Hall the Centre becomes clearly defined as a community facility. It is very much a walk-in neighbourhood building reflecting the scale and local culture of this area, in sharp contrast with the drive-in more hospital-orientated centres as seen in the United States.

The building is comprised of four semi-autonomous sub-buildings arranged around a common circulation area which, in turn, is centred around a courtyard. This concept is carried through into the building interior. The courtyard and circulation routes are treated as soft, informal spaces; the clinical and staff areas are expressed more formally.

The reception area, whilst overlooking the waiting areas, is not directly visible from the main entrance. From reception patients are directed to one of the four waiting zones. Each has a corner play area for children. The zones are defined by a series of timber screens, creating a balance between discreet privacy and isolation from the rest of the building's activities.

The combination of the internal courtyard and the screened waiting zones offers a very relaxed and informal space in which to await consultations. In evaluating the benefits a courtyard can bring to such deep plan arrangements in terms of natural daylight and ventilation, it is surprising that it is not adopted more often.

The proximity of the waiting areas to the consulting rooms whilst reducing travel distance creates the problems of audio confidentiality. This was considered by the architects, who introduced a sound lobby whereby the consulting rooms and waiting areas are separated by two doors. The walls of the clinical block have sufficient mass to cope with sound transmission reduction. Each consulting room is also linked to an interview room via a second sound lobby. This appears to overcome the critical problem of inter-connecting doors often found in primary health care buildings.

It could be argued that such a system of sound lobbies would be cumbersome, especially for the handicapped or elderly patient. However, in practice, once past the first door to the sound lobby the doctor is available to offer assistance within a semi-private zone.

Visual privacy was also taken into consideration. The interior design is deliberately orientated towards the courtyard, with all seats positioned to look on to the courtyard. The incoming daylight and the sculpture as a focal point reinforces this simple, yet subtle interior design.

Within a much wider framework, the basic concept of the courtyard building for primary health care could have other applications and implications. The construction of simple forms centred around a courtyard within the scale of this building has, after all, more to do with the vernacular architecture of the Middle East rather than Northern Europe, yet what it has borrowed (albeit subconsciously) can perhaps be returned to courtyard health centres in hotter climates, utilizing known and local technology (Chapter 5).

The clarity of the plan at Store Heddinge therefore belies an inherent sophistication in the thinking behind the design.

154

Sweden

Population 1990:	**8.31 million**
Percentage of population aged 65 plus 1990:	**17.7**
Population estimated year 2020:	**7.82 million**
Percentage of population aged 65 plus estimated year 2020:	**21.8**
Health care expenditure in pounds per person:	**1002**
Health care expenditure expressed as percentage of GNP:	**8.9**

(Source: Compendium of Health Statistics, Office of Health Economics, London, UK.)

The welfare of Swedish citizens is the responsibility of regional and local government units.

The County Councils (Landsting) govern Sweden at a regional level. Sweden is divided into 24 geographic counties which vary in size and population. Each county is required to provide and administer a co-ordinated health service and medical programme to agreed national standards. To fund such services and programmes councils have the authority to collect taxes from their citizens.

At a local level the municipality (kommun) provides social welfare and care programmes. There are 284 municipalities, each also empowered to levy taxes to support its programmes. Services are also subsidized, if necessary, by central government in order to maintain coherent and consistent standards.

Along with its Scandinavian neighbours, Sweden has traditionally enjoyed high standards of socialized medicine since major social health and welfare programmes were first introduced in the 1940s. Private health care exists on a very limited scale. Only about 5% of physicians are in private practice. The corresponding figure for dentists, however, is more than 50%.

Health care programmes account for 75 to 80% of the total expenditure of most county councils. County council members are directly elected by the population. Among the tasks of these representatives are decisions regarding the economic framework of health care in their area and the size of the county council income tax necessary to finance these activities.

A new Health & Medical Care Act which came into force on 1st January 1983 applies to both medical and health care measures. Under this Act each county council incurs a comprehensive obligation to promote the health of residents in the county council area concerned and to offer them good health care (transport services included) on equal terms. County councils have to plan the development and organization of health and medical care with reference to the aggregate needs of the county population. This planning must also include the health and medical care provided by private practitioners, personnel, medical officers etc.

Although in many respects the county councils operate their health care systems independently, the Swedish state has supervisory powers over these activities. A national health insurance system financed by the state (to a small extent) and by the employers' payroll fees came into being in 1955. Today it provides medical sickness and parental benefits. It covers all Swedish citizens and alien residents.

The health insurance system is mainly an instrument for creating greater social and economic equality. It enables people with small economic resources and/or extensive medical care needs to take advantage of health care services on the same basis as others. Moreover the insurance system functions as a financing instrument, and as an instrument of state control.

The majority of doctors are employed by the county council on a salaried basis. Patients pay a subsidized fee to the county council for each visit to a doctor. The county council is then reimbursed for the balance by the national insurance system.

Until quite recently Swedish medical care had been mainly hospital-orientated. Out-patient care is organized into primary health care districts, each with 5000 to 50,000 inhabitants. Their task is to assume primary responsibility for the health of the population of their area. Each district has one or more local health care centres plus one or more nursing homes for long-term care. At the health centres, district physicians, both general practitioners and specialists provide advisory services and preventive care.

The out-patient system also includes district nurses and district midwives. Ordinarily there are also special centres which provide child health and maternity health care services.

If primary health care resources are insufficient for the measures required for certain diagnostic or treatment programmes, responsibility may be transferred to the county or the regional medical care system.

The Swedish health care system is currently undergoing rapid expansion, and at the same time major changes are taking place in its organizational structure and areas of emphasis. During the past 15 years health service costs have climbed by approximately 15 to 20% annually.

Health care is an important part of the existing Swedish welfare system. The fundamental principle behind it is that all inhabitants should be equally entitled to health care, regardless of where they live in Sweden and what economic resources they have. County councils are responsible for fulfilling this aim. The National Health Insurance System supplements their efforts.

In recent years, health care has attracted increasing attention in the general political debate. This is attributable both to the importance that the health situation of the population occupies in general living standards and to the sharply rising costs of health care.

Among the many objectives to improve access and economic efficiency in the delivery of Sweden's health care system are:

1 To come to grips with the problems of ill health; medical care alone is insufficient. There are growing demands for preventive programmes, including ones that focus on health hazards in the public environment (e.g. the working environment, housing and traffic). Seen from this standpoint, emphasis must be given to an active health policy.
2 The expansion of ambulatory health care outside hospitals (the primary care system) must be given high priority in order to meet demands for proximity, easy access, continuity and quality. Collaboration between this type of out-patient care and the social welfare system also needs to be established.
3 Increased resources are necessary to care for

the chronically ill, especially the elderly, both in their own homes and in local nursing homes.
4 A limit on the number of hospital beds for acute somatic and particularly acute psychiatric care will be necessary. Qualitative reinforcement of psychiatric care is needed, however.
5 Improved nursing care to satisfy the interests of both patients and staff (improved working environment) is an increasingly important demand.
6 In order to provide a balanced development of the health care system, efforts are being made within county councils and elsewhere to improve planning (especially long-term problem- and goal-orientated planning) and to structure health care programmes and resources according to an established model.

These efforts are based on the programmes of principles for health care followed during the 1980s, which the National Board of Health and Welfare worked out during the first half of the 1970s. At the moment, this programme is being reassessed with the aim of developing a new programme on the shape of health care with an eye towards the 1990s.

Following the passing of the Health & Medical Care Acts of 1983 a task force, including politicians and health authorities as well as representatives of labour unions, is empowered to translate the goal of achieving greater access to health care into concrete health policies for the 1990s.

They proposed improvement of primary health care which would be geographically, economically and socially acceptable. As a consequence, additional health centres have been built, to be staffed by general practitioners and nurses. The distribution of financial and other resources between primary, secondary and tertiary care was further reviewed so that more responsibility could be assumed at primary care level. An important co-ordinating force in the improvement of primary care has been the Swedish Planning & Rationalization Institute of the health and social services (SPRI), which was jointly set up in 1968 by the Government and the health care authorities. Its main function since then has been to unravel problems confronting all those who work in the Swedish health sector and to find solutions to promote rationalization. SPRI has also been able to assist Sweden's health services by thinking ahead, foreseeing problems that might arise tomorrow and preparing strategies to tackle them in advance.

The Ekeby Vårdcentral (Health Care Centre)

Location:	**Eskilstuna**
Completed:	**1989**
Type of facility:	**Community health care centre for GP and nursing services with integrated rehabilitation unit**
Architects:	**White Arkitekter AB**
Client:	**Landstinget Sormland Eskilstuna**
Gross floor area:	**1530 sq m (16,500 sq ft)**
Photography:	**Janco Kiellberg**

Architect's statement:

The health care centre at Ekeby mirrors the current trends in Swedish primary health care and is part of Sweden's increased investment in out-patient care, local services and decentralization of specialist out-care. This follows the Swedish Welfare Board's general programme entitled 'Health Care in the 1980s'.

The site is on gently sloping cultivated fields to the south and east, a flat grazing field to the north-east with one or two trees and pine copses to the north. Sparse yew trees and large stone blocks give the area its special character.

The health care centre is situated in a very beautiful location in a large continuous open area comprising fields around Ekeby Farm and the Ekeby gliding field approximately 4 km (2.5 miles) west of the centre of Eskilstuna.

To the west and north-west, the landscape rises and the trees become denser. The entire area is fenced off and is currently grazed by sheep.

To the north of the health care centre lies Ekeby Farm, a delightful old country house finished in traditional red oche wooden panels standing on granite foundations.

The health care centre provides the following accommodation:

- General practitioner surgery
- District nurse's reception including midwifery and child care centres
- Rehabilitation unit comprising physiotherapy, occupational therapy, day health centre (5–10 places) and home health visits.

The most important function of the health care

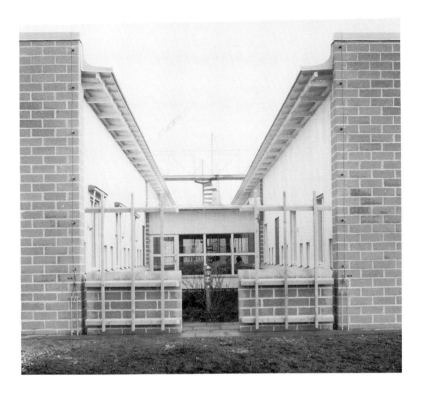

△ *Ekeby Health Care Centre, Ekeby, Eskilstuna.*

centre is to provide local health care services and to work at a local level with the social services and other activities in the health care centre.

The general practitioner's surgery and the district nurse's reception are closely integrated to allow manpower organization according to what is known as the 'health care team principle'.

The centre is divided into two blocks, each containing two sub-departments. Blocks are set at an angle of 20° to each other. An octagonal pavillion links both blocks and also serves as the main entrance. The building volume has been fragmented in this way so that it can harmonize with the area's topographical characteristics.

From the separate access route on the south side of the property are roads leading straight to the main entrance and a walled roundabout for use by taxis and other transport.

Physiotherapy, reception, waiting and staff rooms are located in the south end of the complex. Occupational therapy, day health care, the general practitioner's surgery and the district nurse's office are located in the northern sections.

The interior is characterized by a generous use of natural lighting and quiet, almost sombre colour setting. Doors and corridor floors have different colour markings to facilitate orientation.

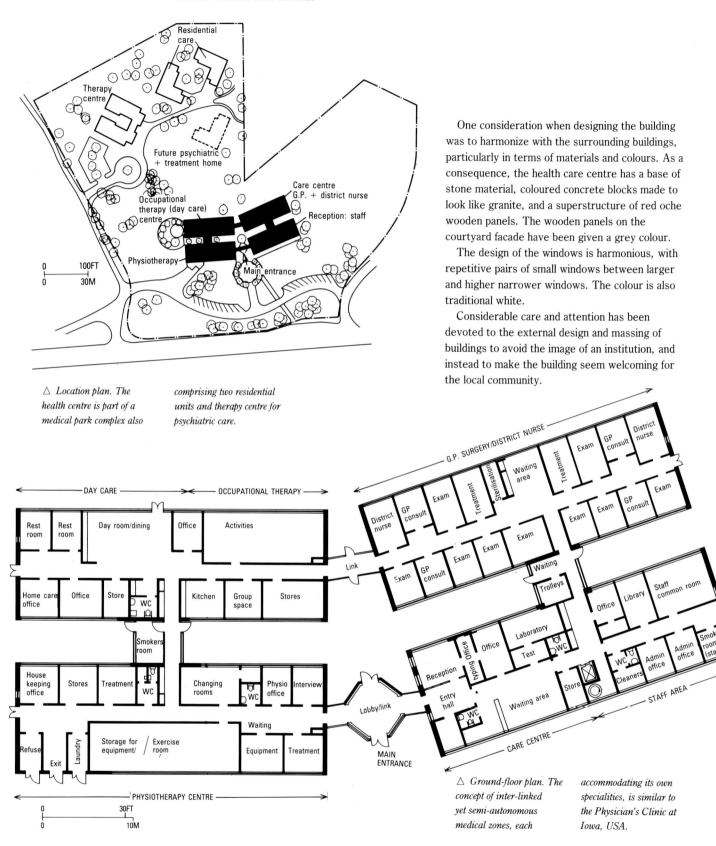

One consideration when designing the building was to harmonize with the surrounding buildings, particularly in terms of materials and colours. As a consequence, the health care centre has a base of stone material, coloured concrete blocks made to look like granite, and a superstructure of red oche wooden panels. The wooden panels on the courtyard facade have been given a grey colour.

The design of the windows is harmonious, with repetitive pairs of small windows between larger and higher narrower windows. The colour is also traditional white.

Considerable care and attention has been devoted to the external design and massing of buildings to avoid the image of an institution, and instead to make the building seem welcoming for the local community.

△ Location plan. The health centre is part of a medical park complex also comprising two residential units and therapy centre for psychiatric care.

△ Ground-floor plan. The concept of inter-linked yet semi-autonomous medical zones, each accommodating its own specialities, is similar to the Physician's Clinic at Iowa, USA.

158

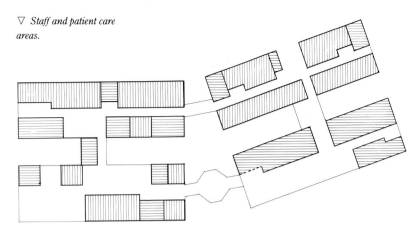

▽ *Staff and patient care areas.*

The pedestrian drive surfaces have different copings. The drive areas are asphalted, whereas the pedestrian and public areas are covered with coloured concrete tiles.

The planted areas and landscaping around the courtyards have been chosen and designed so that they relate to the neighbouring landscape, a landscape that is typical of the county of .Sodermanland, with its characteristic plants and landscape elements. The planted areas around the entrance are made up primarily of broadleafed trees as well as deciduous and evergreen bushes and hedges surrounded by attractive grassed areas.

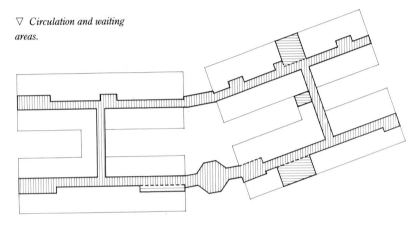

▽ *Circulation and waiting areas.*

Main activity areas

Patients
Dining room
Changing room
Pram store
Waiting (GP/district nurse) (× 3)

Patient care
Nurse room (occupational therapy)
Activities room (occupational therapy)
Group space
Treatment (physiotherapy) (× 2)
Counsellor/interview
Exercise room (physiotherapy)
District nurse
GP consulting (× 4)
Examination (× 9)
Treatment (GP/district nurse) (× 2)

Staff
Therapy office
Home care office
Kitchen
Stores
Housekeeper's office
Physiotherapist's office
Reception

Secretary's office
Laboratory test room
Administration office (× 3)
Staff common room
Staff room for smokers

Comment

The Ekeby Centre is part of a new generation of primary health care facilities that are a result of the re-orientation of the Swedish Health Care Service. Centres such as Ekeby will help to achieve a more balanced position of health buildings which, until recently, were dominated by large and centralized hospital facilities.

As a comparatively new convert to the advantages of a primary health care infrastructure, Sweden has been able to examine and consider its options based upon existing models overseas. It is interesting to note that the Ekeby Centre adopts a

159

▽ *Elevation of centre looking north to physiotherapy wing.*

▷ *View to main entrance which links the two offset wings.*

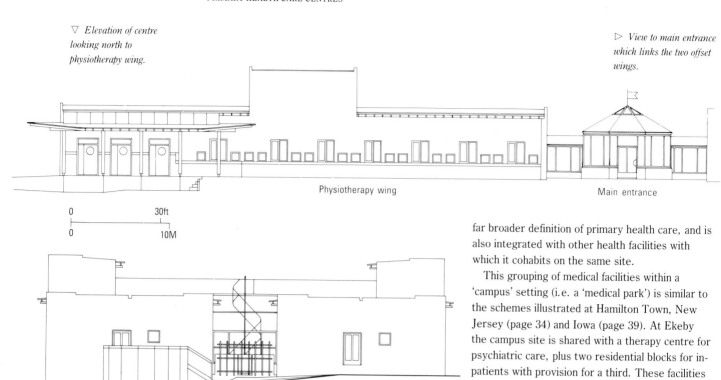

Physiotherapy wing

Main entrance

0   30ft

0   10M

far broader definition of primary health care, and is also integrated with other health facilities with which it cohabits on the same site.

This grouping of medical facilities within a 'campus' setting (i.e. a 'medical park') is similar to the schemes illustrated at Hamilton Town, New Jersey (page 34) and Iowa (page 39). At Ekeby the campus site is shared with a therapy centre for psychiatric care, plus two residential blocks for in-patients with provision for a third. These facilities are also in line with Sweden's desire to move psychiatric care out of hospitals and into the community. The Ekeby site provides a more

Staff area   Courtyard   GP surgery

△ *Elevation of centre looking west to GP's surgery and staff areas.*

▷ *Interior of main entrance hall looking towards the reception and waiting area for the GP surgery.*

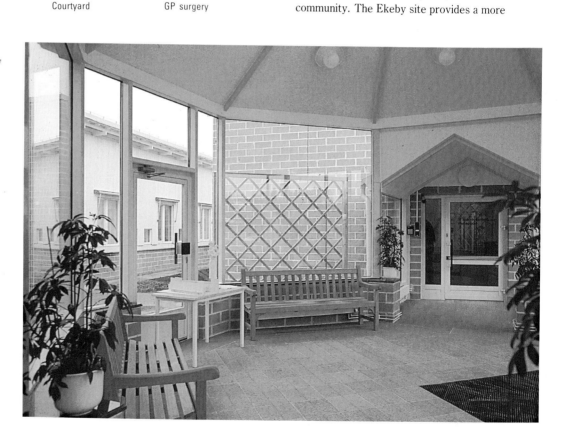

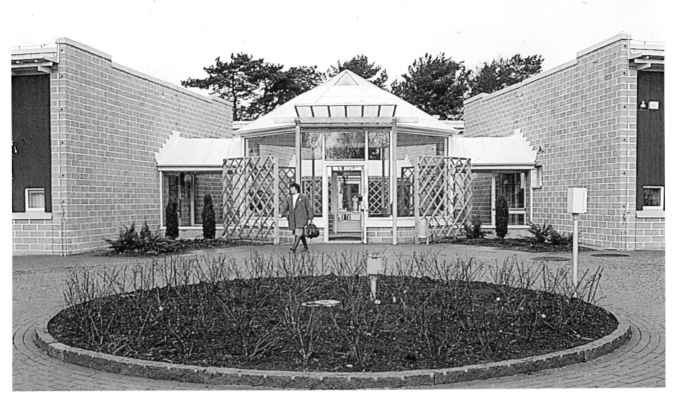

appropriate community environment, and not
hospital-based setting. Too often patients are
discharged to what is loosely defined as 'the
community', without any back-up or structured
support. At Ekeby residents enjoy the benefits of
living within a community setting with the security
of a day care facility available on site.

The centre, conceived and designed as four
units, comprises two blocks connected via a central
link which, in turn, are connected by two further
blocks via an entrance hall and further corridor link.
The design is centred around the philosophy of an
integrated primary health care service. Within one
building there is a general practitioner's surgery
which is also part of a physiotherapy and
occupational therapy day centre.

From the main entrance 'conservatory', visitors
for the doctors or district nurses pass through
reception and then the main waiting area. From
here, visitors pass into a second zone of the care
wing to a waiting area before being directed to see
the doctor or nurse. The nurse and GP work

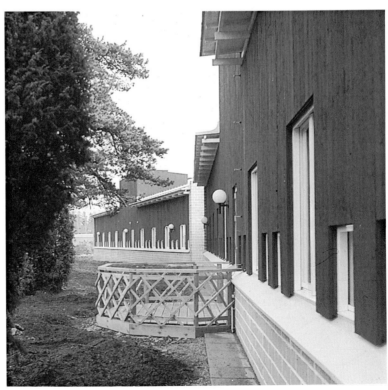

▷ *View to rear of building.*

161

▷ *Side view on to courtyard and central link between the occupational therapy and physiotherapy wings.*

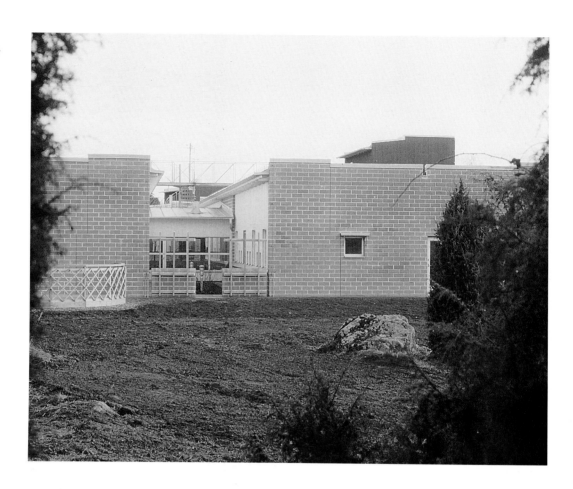

closely together. They are both employed and receive their salary from the county council.

The GP gains access to the therapy wing via a direct circulation link without having to pass through the main entrance.

The other wing functions as a day centre where visitors arrive and may spend several hours involved in physiotherapy or occupational therapy sessions. Included within the day centre is a dining room and patients' rest room.

The concept of linking similar sized modules (as at the Physician's Clinic, Iowa, USA), allows similar and essentially simple forms to be clustered, providing an economical package – repeatable units provide an economy of scale of standardized elements.

The new Swedish health centres appear to embody not just a doctor's surgery concerned with primary medicine, but instead a range of community health and rehabilitation services grouped together to promote a community care service.

The Ekeby Health Care Centre employs these principles and within a very simple and clearly planned layout offers the opportunity for health care staff to work within a collaborative framework. The various zones of the building are clearly defined so that territorial conflicts (as sometimes have occurred in earlier health centres) are avoided. As in international and human relations, co-operation and understanding often take place best within secure and recognized boundaries.

Summary of building projects

In a review of such a diversified cross-section of contemporary primary health care buildings it becomes apparent just how unique each project is, a logical reflection perhaps of a variety of locations, sites, fundings and functional content. There are, however, certain common themes related to the type of building shells which can be described as follows.

Infill/adaption

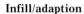

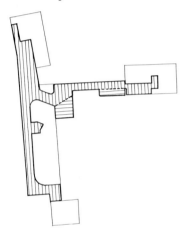

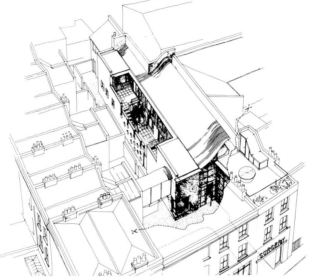

Manor Place, London, UK.

This project was built in response to an existing urban fabric, within which the new surgery had almost to carve out its space requirements. The elongated circulation routes link the centre's disparate parts. The accommodation is located at the end of the circulation 'links' or to one side. There is insufficient space to provide a double-loaded corridor.

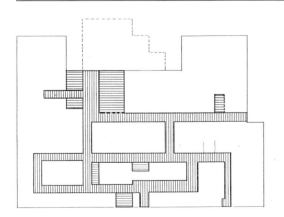

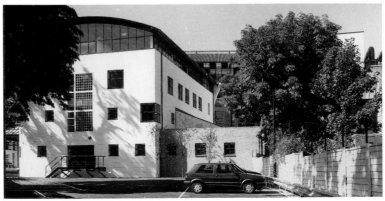

Crowndale Centre, London, UK.

A much larger site and scale of project, yet Crowndale is also a product of urban design engineering. The health centre is merely part of comprehensive care and social service package. The doctors' accommodation is located to one side of a single-loaded corridor; clinic accommodation

163

clusters around the external walls with a corridor link, which in turn surrounds the waiting and health education areas. While this arrangement within a restrictive site allows for natural daylight in the clinical rooms, the waiting and health education areas become internal spaces.

Linear form/double-loaded

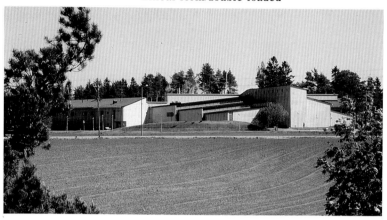

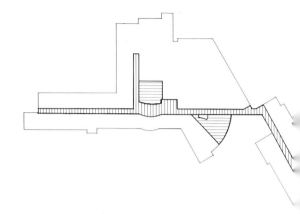

Masku Centre, Masku, Finland.

The accommodation (apart from the deeper plan for the swimming pool) is all accessed from a main circulation route which connects all parts of the building. Rooms are arranged on either side of the corridor offering a comparatively shallow plan and the possibility of natural ventilation. The simplicity of the layout also makes orientation easier for visitors. Special attention was paid to the detail design of the circulation route to alleviate its linear form.

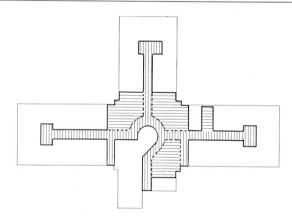

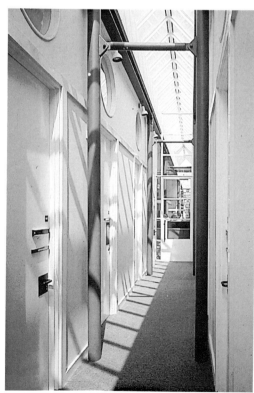

John Telford Clinic, Ilford, UK.

This building is a further refinement of the adaptation of a linear form, utilizing a double-loaded corridor to reduce circulation length. The clinical and staff rooms fan out from a central core containing reception and waiting areas. This arrangement enhances orientation. As with all rooms most pass in and out of the central core. All clinical rooms enjoy natural daylight and ventilation. As a single-storey facility, top-light is introduced to the circulation routes enhancing the environmental quality of the space.

164

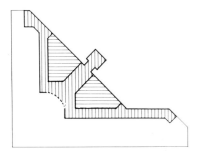

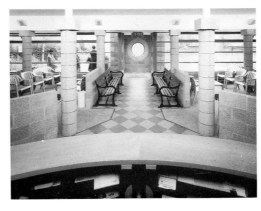

Andover Medical Centre, London, UK.

The triangular plan form is, in many respects, similar to the Lee Bank Health Centre, UK, in that it employs split waiting with the clinical rooms in two zones at right angles to each other. Andover has a simple double-loaded corridor and no race track. Instead the reception/records store is located at the apex of the triangle. As at Store

Heddinge, Denmark, this plan relies upon a detail design which ensures visual and sound privacy from the waiting areas across the corridor to the clinical rooms.

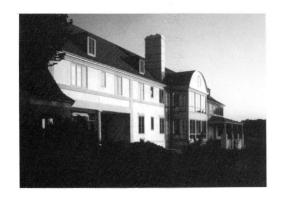

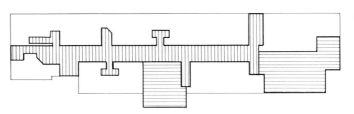

A simple linear plan with single double-loaded corridors running the length of the building. To avoid the monotony of a single and central corridor, the circulation space is fragmented and varied in width, assisting flow past the communal spaces.

Renfrew Center, Pennsylvania, USA.

The spatial quality of this design is that of a country home with circulation areas liberated from the functional chore of connecting one room to another. Instead this building, essentially linear in plan has no definitive corridors, just a series of spaces which flow through one to another. The quality of the building is such that it is most difficult to interpret from a set of plans. The circulation spaces are, however, double-loaded. Both administrative and clinical areas can be accessed.

Highgate Group Practice, London, UK.

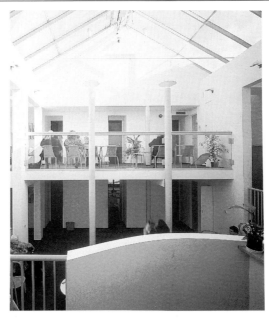

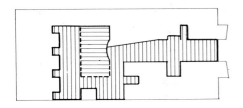

165

The race track

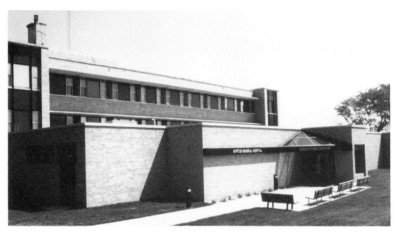

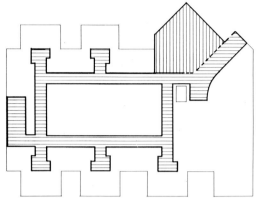

Physician's Clinic, Iowa, USA.

The arrangement is based upon a deep plan with clinical rooms situated to the external walls and treatment spaces grouped in the centre. These are surrounded by the circulation areas on a loop. Internal spaces require artificial ventilation, however in warm climates all accommodation will require air cooling anyway. The central location of the treatment rooms offers across-the-corridor access from the doctors' rooms.

Hamilton Clinic, New Jersey, USA.

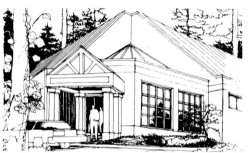

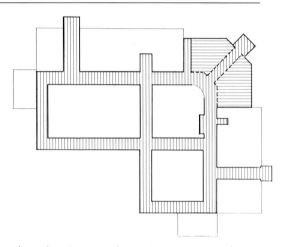

Here the race track is further developed – the circulation route forms three inner cores of rooms with staff and health education areas to either side, to an external wall. Not all the corridor space is double-loaded, yet the plan allows relatively short distances between functional areas. The corridor to the external wall eases orientation, and feeds natural light into other areas. Its juxtaposition to the main entrance node creates symmetry and balance, with functional areas on either side of the diagonal of the main entrance.

Straub Mililani Family Health Care Center, Honolulu, USA.

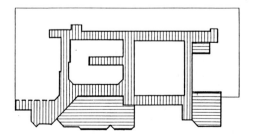

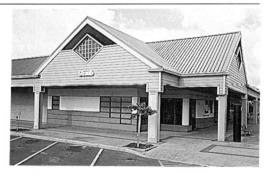

The plan has two central core areas: treatment and nursing stations. The treatment room conveniently services the examination rooms and is also adjacent to the nursing station. The race track concept applies, with the main circulation surrounding these

166

two core service areas. The more cellular accommodation (i.e. examination rooms) is positioned at the rear, off a double-loaded corridor.

At each end of the building are larger, more interconnected staff areas, staff rooms and reception filing zones.

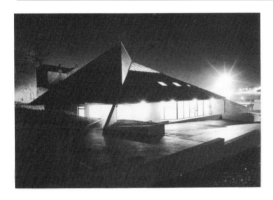

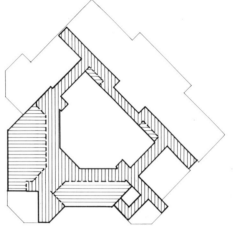

Bridge Street Medical Centre, Belfast, UK.

Off the entrance, the waiting areas are split and linked via the circulation route to the respective clinical rooms. The plan allows separate practices to operate independently under one roof. Common staff areas are centrally located and surrounded by the circulation routes (the race track). Each clinical

area located on the other side of the race track is naturally lit and ventilated. Daylight also penetrates the central staff court by top-lighting.

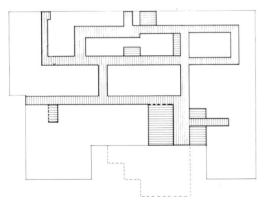

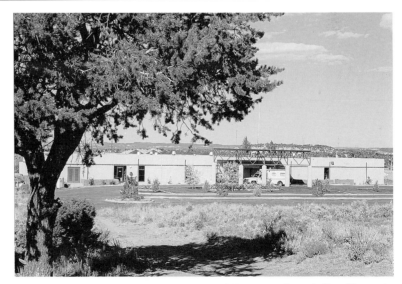

As with the Hamilton Clinic, New Jersey, USA, Inscription House has essentially three inner cores, around which the circulation routes run. The three core areas comprise a laboratory and health record store, emergency treatment and nursing station screening. The building is zoned to take account of its multi-use facility, that is, field health, physical therapy, dental, emergency and clinical uses. The design team paid particular attention to combining

the opportunities for an effective, and essentially contemporary building envelope, with due regard to the specific cultural requirements of its user population.

Inscription House Health Center, Arizona, USA.

167

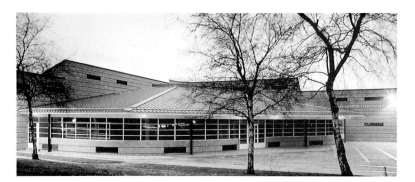

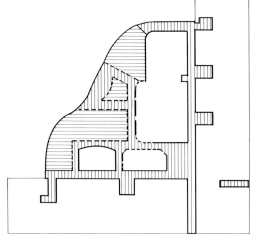

Lee Bank Health Centre, Birmingham, UK.

A very similar plan to the Bridge Street Medical Centre, with waiting areas again split, and staff/ reception/records forming the central core around which runs the circulation route. Corridors are double-loaded so that the clinical areas forming the two perimeter zones are within easy access to records and reception. These, in turn, overlook the public spaces of entrance and waiting.

Store Heddinge Medical Centre, Stevns, Denmark.

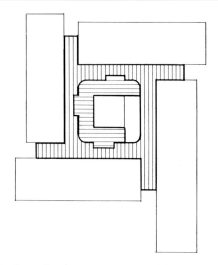

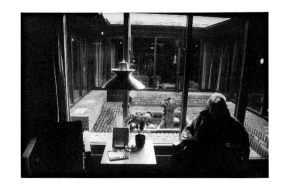

The Store Heddinge plan developed the race track concept providing a building that appears almost as a 'catherine wheel' revolving around its central courtyard. Waiting areas are planned deep inside the facility, but with the introduction of an internal courtyard these enjoy daylight and natural ventilation. The plan relies, however, upon provision of visual and audio privacy from the waiting areas to the clinical rooms. As at the Ekeby Centre, Sweden, repeated plan forms are exploited and crafted to create a highly sophisticated, yet simple, design solution to a complex set of functional constraints.

Deep plan/double-loaded circulation

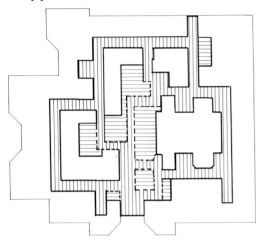

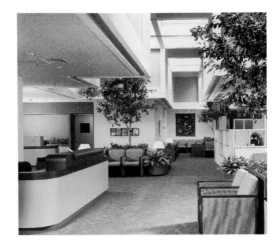

Valley Forge Health Center, Philadelphia, PA, USA.

The fitting out of a commercial building shell as at Valley Forge necessitates maximum use of the existing space available. Here clinical rooms are arranged to the perimeter with clusters of treatment facilities surrounded by the major circulation route. Waiting areas are internal and all spaces require artificial lighting, cooling and ventilation.

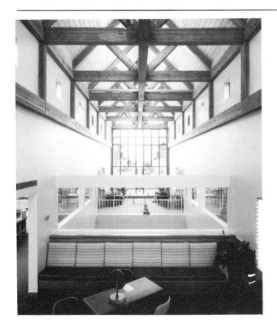

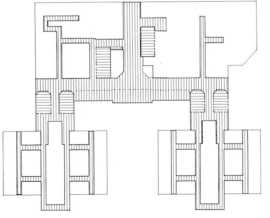

Rockwood Clinic, Portland, Oregon, USA.

The double-loaded corridor feeds into both deep plan and perimeter-based spaces. The concept is based upon a module, two per floor, each connected to the main service and entrance areas.

Such repetition of units offers an economy of scale in the design and construction procurement. In each module the doctors' rooms are located with benefit from the external walls, examination, treatment and nursing stations are located deep in the plan. Waiting areas are clustered at the entrance to each module. The circulation areas within the main service and entrance blocks become a focal point of the Center for all visitors entering and leaving the building.

169

Linear plan/double-loaded circulation

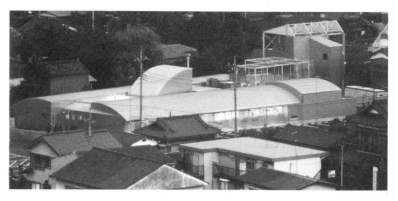

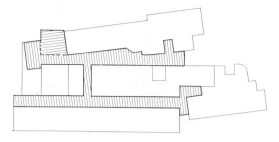

Harayama Clinic, Tohgane, Japan.

The centre is arranged as three functional zones with two circulation routes running in parallel the length of the building, and a further corridor to link the three zones. The internal functional zone accommodates the mainly surgical/treatment procedures, and the two outer zones accommodate patient bedrooms, waiting and reception and doctors' rooms. Each zone therefore relates to a specific function, with the inner treatment zone equally accessible to the other two.

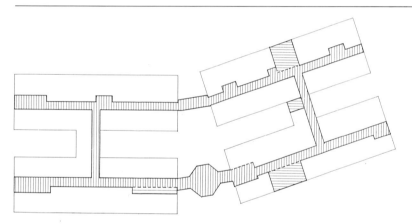

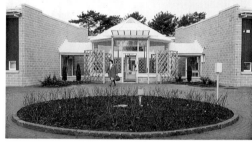

Ekeby Centre, Eskilstuna, Sweden.

The concept of two parallel corridors is continued at Ekeby. The Centre is actually made up of two separate buildings, circulation routes form the link and the main entrance. Each building is, in turn, further divided into two zones with a single corridor linking the two. The use of open-ended internal courtyards brings daylight and natural ventilation to each of the functional rooms which open off the double-loaded corridors.

Architecture for Primary Health Care: a wider perspective

Health care expenditure expressed as percentage of gross national profit (GNP)

1987 figures	% GNP	Compared with average of OECD countries (8.4%)	Percentage change 1977–87	Compared with average percentage change in OECD countries (18%)
Denmark	6.7	−1.7	−8	−26
Finland	6.7	−1.7	−3	−21
Japan	5.2	−3.2	+2	−16
Sweden	8.9	−0.5	+7	−11
UK	5.8	−2.6	+12	−6
USA	11.1	+2.7	+25	+7

Health care expenditure in £ per person (1987)

	Health care expenditure	Compared with average of OECD countries (885)	Percentage change 1977–87	Compared with OECD average change (+60%)
Denmark	777	−208	−4	−64
Finland	732	−153	+31	−33
Japan	625	−260	+189	+120
Sweden	1002	+117	−5	−65
UK	423	−462	+41	−19
USA	1252	+367	+51	−19

Populations

	Population 1990 (million)	% of population aged 65+	Population estimated 2020 (million)	% of population aged 65+
Denmark	5.12	15.4	4.80	21.2
Finland	4.97	13.0	5.04	19.9
Japan	123.87	11.4	132.61	20.8
Sweden	8.31	17.7	7.82	21.8
UK	56.19	15.6	56.08	17.8
USA	248.43	12.2	304.36	15.4

Summary tables for countries as discussed in case studies.

Source for health care expenditure is International Monetary Fund (IMF). Source for statistics:

Compendium of Health Statistics, 7th edn, Office of Health Economics, London, UK, 1989.

A recurring international theme is that hospitals are far too predominant in health services. Yet the extension of primary care is not normally associated directly with a reduction in specialized care at hospitals, even though certain programmes clearly report a surplus in capacity of this form of care.

Long-term care is an exception to the general move towards limiting in-patient care. Indeed, an increase in the number of beds for long-term care will be necessary. There is, however, a strong desire in the health service planning of different countries to extend primary care. This was especially noticeable in Finland following the introduction of the Public Health Act 1972. In general the importance of primary care focusing on preventive measures and health education is emphasized, as is the need for greater co-operation between doctors and other categories of staff, and between medical care and social welfare. Finally, there is a need for citizens to have a greater influence over the forms of primary care.

Primary health care is not an unequivocal concept. It can be interpreted from either a functional or organizational point of view. As can be seen from the case studies, views on what is encompassed by 'primary care' can also vary from one country to another.

Most of the tasks of primary care in the majority of Western European countries are dealt with by private practitioners. In many of these countries – such as Great Britain, Ireland, The Netherlands, Austria and Denmark – primary care is controlled through political decisions concerning that country's health services. In other countries – such as the United States, Japan, Italy and Belgium – it is the private practitioners who decide on the emphasis and localization of activities. Patient charges and private health insurance schemes are of great importance in these forms of care.

In many countries, nurses are being trained so that they will be able to perform more of the tasks that have hitherto been carried out by doctors. In Canada and the United States, for example, nurses can undergo specialist training to become nurse-practitioners. A similar development is becoming increasingly apparent in the United Kingdom, particularly in medical screening and health information with certain categories of nurses performing increasingly independent and more qualified tasks. All these rely upon suitable building environments in which to allow such progress and change to happen.

It is encouraging to witness (as demonstrated in the case studies) the strength of dialogue between architecture and medicine. Each needs the other to create an appropriate environment for the effective delivery of health care in that community. Hospitals, because of their sheer scale of facilities, tend to lead to large and often impersonal buildings. In such cases the architect's client will not necessarily be the primary end-user. Opportunities for reflecting the subtleties and philosophies of the medical practitioners within the building design are rare and often buried under the weight of administrative procedures.

However, when the bureaucracy and anonymity of the client body is stripped away, as becomes possible in primary health care buildings, a highly focused and articulate client is revealed. It is possible for the architect to become far more sensitized to the needs and requirements of the building users, both staff and patients. In the United States many HMO programmes have encouraged greater architectural input to offer a more personalized image of medical care. Architecture can therefore play a greater role in projecting the image of primary health care. This is an important factor, not only for centres that rely upon capitation-related income, but also to support and encourage preventive and health education programmes. In this way, architecture plays a part in the overall marketing and care programme strategy of the United States' HMO and investor-owned hospital organizations.

The architecture of primary health care is related to human scale and sensitivity. It is about reassurance, trust and the relationship between the patient and medical practitioner. It is neither a monument to the institution of medicine, nor architecture.

Clinics have been forced by competition and consumer preferences to move away from stainless steel metal doors, linoleum, insensitive lighting and bland institutional colour schemes. The emphasis on 'high-touch' means the physician-administrators are asking their architectural consultant to help them de-institutionalize, de-stress and dress up their waiting rooms, clinics and hospital service areas. Along with this there is an emphasis on communication and patient circulation.
Dr John W. Grigsby, physician, Portland, USA. Busker,

G. (1987) Architecture as an asset in health care. *Architecture*, January, p. 3).

The building environment of primary health care centres does not imply necessarily that the setting is domestic. Patients have the right to remain anonymous to all except their medical, professional and appropriate support staff. A balance between environments that are warm and welcoming but also efficient and discreet, where information exchange and one's own body is treated in confidence and with discretion, has to be achieved.

Primary health care is not just concerned with medicine. It encompasses a far broader range of activities from health education to counselling. The environments to accommodate this broad spectrum therefore need to flex and respond almost at once to such a diverse and essentially unpredictable range of functions.
Derek Salter, Care Design Group

The case studies indicate that both private and socialized medicine are in a period of transition towards more consumer-based health care services. The institutionalization of care is perceived as patronizing, and therefore new forms of environment that de-institutionalize and dispense with the paternalistic connotations of architecture for medicine are being explored. This does not automatically imply a 'cosy domestic' approach to design.

There are many examples of primary care design, particularly in the United Kingdom, which have sought refuge behind a pseudo vernacular domestic facade. This domestication of medical architecture is, as John Allan has suggested, in part a reflection of the renewed distrust of technological medicine. Yet isn't the misuse of domestic architecture patronizing in itself?

Yet the case studies have shown that when there is a freshness of thought and a confidence based upon a real awareness of the physical and emotional needs of the users, opportunities are created for excellence in architecture for primary health care.

What lessons can be learned to detect those trends which will shape the demand for primary health care buildings in the 1990s and into the next century: our futures?

An international perspective

The United States

In the private medical financial systems of the United States primary health care services will become more accountable to the patient. Private medicine relies upon numbers and in primary care in particular attracting as many patients to take part in health screening, education and preventive medicine sessions for such programmes to be effective.

Far more attention and resources will be paid to creating environments for the needs of the patient, rather than just the medical staff.

The quality of the facilities themselves will increasingly become a major marketing tool.
Joe Jordan, WRT Architects

In primary health care, which tends to present the medical world's broadest frontier as the general population, the image of the patient is being refocused. Rather than the patient being viewed as the grateful receiver of medical care, the patient has become the purchaser and consumer of health and medical services. This wave of consumer awareness has reached both architecture and medicine. Through perhaps a greater awareness generated particularly in the United States, patients can no longer be perceived as passive recipients of health care but rather as active participants.

In medical care (assuming adequate health insurance cover) choice may not necessarily be exercised as a result of the cost of service but the quality and type of environment from which those services are delivered.

Architecture and interior design is therefore being viewed, particularly in the United States, as a key player in the promotion of that image to its patients/clients. The architect is moving across from the building to the marketing team. Good quality and sensitive design become important factors in communicating a facility's public image and in promoting its services.
Derek Salter, Care Design Group

As health care in the United States becomes more orientated towards primary health care provision, so the importance of appropriate architectural design is underlined, simply because of the higher through-put of patients and the power of choice.

Major problems lie ahead in the United States regarding the affordability of health services. It is widely accepted that the present system of a largely private health service is inequitable and inefficient. There appears little scope in the short term to improve matters. The budgetary burden of extending insurance to those without cover is regarded as prohibitive. Health care costs for operators and consumers continue to escalate.

As hospital organizations attempt to diversify because of a drop in patient loads this also provides more opportunities for the development of a more consumer-orientated primary health care service.

Lynn Bonge, of the Omaha-based architectural firm of Henningson Durham & Richardson, in an article in the February 1987 edition of *Building Design & Construction* stated that

In a community that had four or five viable hospitals five years ago, today three probably will be profitable, one will be just getting by and one will be forced to close. Hospitals' emphasis in the near future will be on ambulatory care facilities. Some may be built at more accessible sites than their current locations and could become a nucleus for medical malls that might include life care facilities.[1]

However, the fundamental challenge of America's future health system will be its method of financing. While some prefer to place the responsibility of insurance cover on employers, this will only increase the burden upon smaller companies and could well result in reducing staff and increasing the proportion of those Americans without employment or health cover. Washington has looked to European models of universal health care, working alongside the current market economy of medical services. Community-based health services will therefore move increasingly towards the centre stage of the political debate. The challenge of America's health future will be to research and explore ways to provide a more equitable means of health care provision for all.

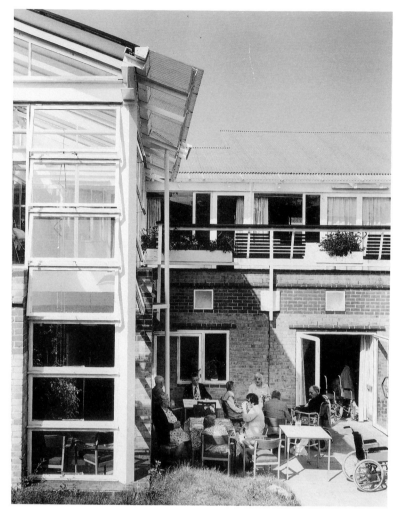

△ *The Lambeth Community Care Centre patients enjoying their lunch together, organized by the patients for both their staff and their staff's enjoyment symbolizing the independent philosophy of the Centre. Architect: Edward Cullinan. Photography: Martin Charles*

- Speech therapy
- Chiropody
- Dentistry
- Medical and nursing care

The concept of a community-based health care facility for the provision of health care and treatment has its roots in the innovative models of the Peckham and Finsbury Health Centres of the 1930s (page 5). As at Finsbury, such innovation by the user group/client is matched by its architectural solution. The architects, Edward Cullinan, worked alongside the client group to develop the brief and have captured in the building the spirit of what is a radical health care facility built against the grain of decreasing state-funded health care expenditure.

In 1985, *Architect's Journal* gave detailed coverage of the building in terms of its design, user requirement and costs.[2] Such information is therefore not repeated in this book, however the building's significance lies once again in the theme of architecture and medicine, and how inspired and progressive this dialogue can be if each has the confidence to allow (or risk) the other to play a creative role and so advance the state of the art. Edward Cullinan as architect in discussing the brief invited the client to think in terms of activities and functions, and not simply forms. Because the funding and users came from a variety of authorities and departments, the architects had to steer the discussions away from the traditional way of thinking towards a view of the centre as a whole. The centre was blessed with a highly articulate and in many ways equally radical client group who responded to the community architecture approach of Edward Cullinan and his team, resulting in a totally refreshing example of community-based health care facilities.

A further trend towards a more integrated framework of planning primary health care services was initiated by the Government's White Paper 'Promoting Better Health' (CM 249 1987).[3] If the objectives of the White Paper are achieved this could well overcome the current disparity of

The United Kingdom

From a largely state funded and controlled health service, recent developments in the 1990s have shifted accountability of the National Health Service towards more locally-based managers. There is fierce public debate as to the future of the National Health Service. However, there appears to be consensus that health services should respond more to patients' needs in terms of services and facilities.

A worthy example of user/client participation resulting in a facility which meets local needs is the Lambeth Community Care Centre completed in 1985. The care centre provides 20 in-patient beds, a 35 place day centre and a medical facility which includes the following health care services:

- Physiotherapy
- Occupational therapy

174

standards and the very fragmented nature of primary health care premises throughout the United Kingdom.

As in the United States, the patients are being encouraged to exercise their choice as consumers of patient primary health care services. New arrangements offer patients the ability to choose and change their general practitioner, subject to the patient being within the doctor's catchment area.

In turn general practitioners are now being encouraged to promote their health care services and, in effect, compete within a newly created market place of primary health care. Financial incentives will also encourage a broader range of services, including the undertaking of minor surgical procedures. This will no doubt benefit the patient and remove the pressure for services from hospitals; however the undertaking of such procedures will rely upon adequate and appropriate facilities. If the patient (as consumer) demands these services, so the provision of facilities will need to respond to this demand.

In an attempt to exert greater financial control over the cost of primary health care, GPs are also being asked by central government to be more accountable in the running of their primary health care services. A shift away from revenue for GPs is also taking place, that is, away from direct reimbursement on a capitation basis to a fee-for-service system, though it is intended that patients will still receive service free of charge at the point of delivery. Therefore a greater proportion of general practitioners' income will relate to the range of services that can be offered.

The above factors will shape and influence the type of buildings needed to accommodate future primary health care services. If the patient has the power of choice, so the quality of the environment and its range of facilities will tend to be a reflection of this choice. Good architecture becomes a marketing tool, the public face of an efficient and well-organized primary health care centre.

Yet while the underlying trend is to improve premises, greater control is being exercised by the Government over the amount of available funds

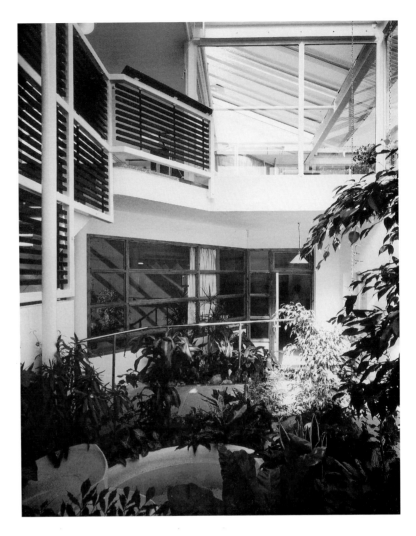

under National Health Insurance provision. From 1990 budgets for general practitioner premises (both improvements and new build) became cash limited. Notwithstanding a radical change in the country's economic fortunes, it appears unlikely that strict controls of capital expenditure budgets will relax significantly under different political regimes.

Such chronic capital underfunding is forcing GPs to explore alternative forms of financing better premises or simply delay the building projects until state funding becomes available.

In October 1992 a report into London's health service (known as the Tomlinson Report) was published, which actually recommended the closure of a number of London's hospitals and for funding to be increased instead for improved primary and community health care premises and services.[4]

△ *The Lambeth Community Care Centre view on to the Centre's two-storey conservatory creating a therapeutic environment. The Lambeth Community Care Centre is an innovative and refreshing project, but is it a 'swan song' of Great Britain's publicly-funded health care culture, or perhaps a glimpse of a better future? Architect: Edward Cullinan. Photography: Martin Charles*

Sweden

Despite a high level of state funded health care, Sweden is a relative newcomer to primary health care, yet it has tabled an agenda for greater emphasis to be placed upon community rather than hospital-based health care.

The Swedish Planning & Rationalization Institute of the health and social services (SPRI) published a report entitled 'Primary Care in Progress' in 1984. This set out the objectives for developing primary health care services in Sweden for the 1990s and beyond. Included in its recommendations were the promotion of primary health care by:

- a unified primary care organization within every county council
- the development of more concrete goals and objective of primary care
- measures to improve conformity between political goals and practical programmes within primary care.[5]

According to the SPRI, primary care will also need to co-operate with other parts of the health and medical care system. Primary care and county medical care should complement each other. In order for society to realize maximum benefits from specialized hospital care, expanded primary care services are needed which can then deal with everyday health problems. Among other things, such services would relieve a large part of the hospital's out-patient care responsibilities as well as in the long term decreasing the need for in-patient care.

Primary care is also required in communities with hospitals as they do not satisfy the same kinds of needs for care. Proximity to a hospital does not provide a guarantee that care is easily accessible. Continuity of care is often neglected in hospitals. Likewise, specialized care does not provide the opportunity of dealing with the comprehensive nature of the patient's primary care needs. Thus primary care has an important role to fulfil even in communities served by hospital services.

The need for care increases with an increasing number of elderly people. There are two essential questions, however – can their needs be met and how can elderly people's own desires be fulfilled. There is a significant risk that elderly people will become caught, institutionalized in patient care and eventually be hospitalized. Primary care can offer alternative forms of health care and serve to co-ordinate medical and social resources (for example, nursing at home, nursing at day care centres and home-maker services). These provide benefits that are humanitarian, care-orientated and economic.

Significant continued development of primary care can be accomplished through organizational methods, educational and information resources with increased co-ordination. Relatively small economic sacrifices will probably be required. The economic contribution which is necessary, however, will probably have to be achieved through the re-organization of Sweden's health and medical care resources. This will not necessarily mean that a sufficient level of resources for hospital activities will be at risk. Primary care (excluding nursing homes) represents at present less than 10% of Sweden's total operational expenses. An acceptable level for development of primary care will only require a marginal increase in this figure.

It is therefore important to recognize the advantages of primary care and the unique possibilities it can offer to the community. At the same time it is also important to point out that the discussion concerning potential primary care must be refined as long as significant variations exist regarding the level of development.

The Swedish model of primary health care is developing within a far broader definition of care. In recent years Sweden, along with other Scandinavian countries, has as a result of political initiatives achieved a substantial shift of resources away from hospitals towards community-based medical care. A typical example is the community health care centre at Upplands, Vasby, near Stockholm. This is physically integrated into a shopping mall and contains long-term residential accommodation for 40 elderly people, together with a health centre and an extensive range of services.

As illustrated with the Ekeby Centre (page 157), primary health care buildings may also include day care facilities for physiotherapy and occupational therapy. Sweden has made a commitment to improve its primary health care facilities. Despite increasing financial constraints on a largely state-funded health care system, it is set to increase the proportion of health expenditure in this field, albeit at the expense of the already well-developed hospital infrastructure. It could well prove to be an important arena for future innovation.

Finland

Finland was nominated as a pilot country for 'health for all by the year 2000' by the World Health Organisation. The Primary Health Care Act of 1972 set down targets for improvements in the network of primary care, many of which have now been achieved. As illustrated at the Masku Centre (page 139), primary care is broadly defined with in-patient accommodation seen as an integrated part of a primary health care network of facilities. As Finland continues to reinforce a strong commitment to primary health care, the community-based health centre will play an increasing role. The aim is for all communes and communal federations to establish health centres. These are to include physicians, consultation services, emergency services, an ambulance service, health education for children, mothers and adults, school health care services as well as in some cases occupational health and dental care.

The health centres will also aim to treat minor mental disorders and after a psychiatric patient has been discharged from a special hospital to take on the responsibility of follow-up treatment in collaboration with a mental health centre. The target is integration of psychiatric health care with other sectors of health care.

Increasingly essential forms of service in health centres will have, besides the actual ward services, supervised home care and day hospital services. The health centre wards will aim to care for

patients requiring acute primary health care or follow-up treatment, and long-term patients not suited to home care (see Masku Centre, page 139). Finland's objectives will be to integrate the various community and primary care services, to secure health care and medical treatment programmes that are as versatile as possible and located close to population centres.

Denmark

In Denmark the system of health centres will continue to provide the basis for the delivery of its primary health care. The expensive hospital will lead to a continued emphasis on this programme. The nature of a fragmented and locally-based health provision is suited to the small and often remotely located populations of Denmark. Yet in common with other European countries, and the United States, the increasing number of elderly people will place an increasing load on the community and health care services. With a diminishing number of carers, the ability for elderly people to be cared for in their own homes may over-stretch the staff and resources of community-based nurses. This implies an expanding role for primary health care centres to work alongside community care agencies.

The relative stability of Denmark's state-funded health care system and those in other Scandinavian countries will therefore need to prepare for a population that is becoming increasingly 'top heavy' in terms of its age profile. This will inevitably place greater demands upon the health service, particularly in community-based, primary care and long-term care services. The problem on the horizon could be the diminishing pool of workers who will, through direct or indirect taxation, be called upon to fund the additional facilities and resources that will be required. Some have argued that long-term care insurance, although an American phenomenon, may have to be considered so that the working population can contribute to their own long-term care after retirement.

177

Japan

Through science and technology, Japan has eradicated many of the tropical epidemics that afflicted its population in the past. Its primary health care future is now similar to those in Western cultures: health screening for heart conditions, health education for better dietary habits, etc.

The circumstances of Japanese health are changing. The highly aged society, the transition of the disease structure from communicable diseases to chronic diseases and the innovation of health care demand now place new demands on health care in Japan. As for primary health care, the health services for the aged and the mentally handicapped will be the most important problems to be solved, while at the same time an efficient and effective health care supply system will need to be further established.

Through government legislation there is now a greater emphasis on services for older people required and allowed for within health centres. With the problems of mental frailty is the need to provide facilities for the treatment and care of senile dementia, which is seen as one of the most serious problems in Japan's ageing society.

As in Finland, mental health will be based within the community with health centres and mental health centres co-ordinating mental health activities, allowing patients to move within the community, rather than being based in centralized institutions.

A wider perspective: Eastern Europe

Events of the last decade in Eastern Europe and the former Soviet republics, will, among many other factors, have ramifications on most country's health services in both the medium and long term.

The combination of changes to the social/political systems, combined with the new voice of consumers of health services may well lead to the evolution of new forms of primary health care services. Socialized medicine, as operated in Scandinavia, may well be the preferred method, but this relies upon a high percentage of personal taxation. Private medical plans, however, are still a possibility with the evolving plural market economies of the former Eastern Block.

Third and fourth worlds

The poor nations of the world, caught in a vicious circle of malnutrition and disease are, of course, in urgent need of aid and support. Through the admirable work of the World Health Organization and other international agencies, further advances are being made towards the WHO goal of 'health for all by the year 2000'.

The concept of primary health care as a community-based and essentially low-tech infrastructure for health promotion and illness prevention is, perhaps, a more appropriate framework of support than the import of westernized medicine and technology within hospitals.

Support in primary health care facilities should allow appropriate and indigenous technology and medical expertise to develop, respecting the autonomy of culture as an integral part of health care. There is much that the communities of the world can learn from each other. The death of an individual from hunger is a tragedy, yet so is the unnecessary death caused by the failure of a person's heart due to excessive cholesterol and high fat foods. It is within such extremes of world affluence and poverty that primary health care can play an increasingly important role for future generations.

While attention and financial resources are quite rightly required in Third World countries there are also the inhabitants of the Fourth World. These are the deprived and run-down inner city areas of often quite prosperous First World centres. Primary care in major cities such as London, Birmingham, Washington, New York, etc. suffer from a chronic lack of medical staff and facilities. The provision of adequate facilities is therefore a major problem.

Existing doctors' surgeries have tended to out-grow their original premises; local populations are often those in most need of primary care services. Yet there is limited land upon which to build. Even when sites are identified, they are prohibitively expensive. Further hurdles are sometimes erected by planning/zoning authorities. Because such premises tend to be small, they often inhibit the growth of primary care services, with doctors tending to work on their own (single handed) without a team for support. The workload of the single-handed inner city doctor offers little or no opportunity for health education and preventive medical programmes.

In London the plight of primary health care in the inner cities was highlighted by the Jarman Report[6] following that of the Acheson Report[7] (both 1981). These reports also drew attention to the significant number of inner city GPs who are approaching or past retirement age, and the need to encourage young doctors to enter general practice in the inner city. While the availability of land is still a major problem in London at least health authorities are now opening dialogues with planning and zoning authorities to create a more positive platform on which to build primary health care facilities. The Crowndale and Andover centres (pages 120 and 128) are witnesses to this, though there is still much work to be done.

An ageing population: care in the community
Nearly 11% of the world's urbanized population is aged 65 and over. Throughout all major industrialized countries there is an increasing 'age wave', that is, an increasing proportion of elderly people in relation to other age groups.

This shift in the demographic balance of the population is therefore largely a universal phenomenon. The increasing numbers of elderly people will bring greater demands upon social and health support services. Apart from prohibitive costs of long-term care in hospitals, it is of course beneficial to allow elderly people to be cared for in their own homes or at least within a community care setting. As Laing and Buisson report

The most likely scenario for the 1990s is a more rapid shift towards primary care than the trend scenario would suggest. New pressures to develop ambulatory care will rise in response to cost pressures and consumer expectations.[8]

Care in the community programmes, as proposed by the United Kingdom Government, will further encourage this trend from institutional to community-based care. However, these programmes will, to a large extent, rely upon adequate primary health care facilities and funding.

It will also require integration of primary health care services within the local network of other community-based care services and facilities such as nursing homes and day centres (secondary care).

New links between secondary and primary care are likely to be created and there will be a shift in culture towards prevention. The 'health enterprise' of the 1990s will have greater integration between hospital and community services, earlier discharge and more day treatment and with greater emphasis on health promotion.[9]

A new approach to primary health care services can also be seen within changing medical and health definitions of patient treatment, that is, treating the patient as a whole person and not just the illness.

The new age health centre
A definite trend to creating a facility that does not represent a technical approach to medicine but instead embraces and supports the well-being of the patient as a whole can be foreseen. This of course follows a greater sense of humanism that has developed in post-modern architecture, that is a contrast with the technically driven ideas of previous decades.
Joe Jordan

As reported in the American Institute of Architecture's 'Memo' (September 1990) entitled *Vision 2000: Health Care Design*, Donald McKahan of Lennon Associates writes:

A more holistic paradigm of medicine will re-unite body and mind with both a high-tech and high-touch approach to health care. The hospital 'body shop' of the 1980s will give way to a new era of health centers designed to harness the mind's potential through the visualization techniques of healing imagery.[10]

Our health is inextricably linked to the way we live our lives and to how we protect and care for our planet. The problems of global warming through pollution and the breakdown of the earth's protective barriers will affect the health and, ultimately, the survival of all life forms for generations to come. Consciousness of the need to protect our planet is, however, beginning to develop world-wide, in recognition of the need to preserve our natural resources for future generations. This helps us understand the shift towards a new medical era in which the role of drugs and surgery (unnatural and limited resources) will diminish, and the role of medicine becomes part of a wider health issue. Many primary health care doctors (in particular the British Association for Holistic Medicine in London and the American Holistic Medical Association in North Carolina) are recognizing the benefits of using complementary therapies which help to reduce the use of costly drugs or invasive surgery. With the recognition that our health is linked to our surroundings comes the need to create a healthy environment. Primary health care centres can themselves be part of this new era in which buildings offering health care are designed in the knowledge that we are linked not only to nature but also to the materials used to house us.

One possible future direction is the more holistic approach to primary and community care found in the Blackthorn Trust Medical Centre in Maidstone, Kent. Architects David Sutherland and Wolodymyr Radysh of Camphill Architects, Aberdeen, Scotland, have described their approach to this new centre:

It has long been recognized that the organic approach to architecture is a response to the human need for forms that have an obvious relationship to nature and have a direct connection to the earth. In a mechanistic age which has seen great advances in technology, buildings tend towards an expression governed by a rectilinear form. Organic architecture has been shunned because invariably forms result from a different way of thinking and different fundamental beliefs.

The three doctor NHS practice in Maidstone, added artistic therapies to their practice as a means of being more effective in healing the patients, many of whom have chronic illnesses, difficult to cure by conventional methods. Art therapy was initially met with scepticism, but soon clearly proved to be an important asset.

Eurythmy (a form of therapeutic movement) was introduced along with therapeutic modelling, music and counselling. The relationship between the respective therapists and group of doctors developed naturally into team work where together they could share and assess the diagnoses, prescribe medication, including therapies and could review progress. The team approach became the absolute strength and foundation of the practice, at the heart of which was a shared understanding of the human being, not only as a physical being but as having a soul and spirit which work quite specifically into a physical body. This picture of a man or woman as described by Rudolph Steiner forms the basis of a complete, artistic approach to healing. It also requires a deep understanding of the uniqueness of each individual patient.

The new building to continue and expand this innovative field of work, which reflected the healing approach and the community practice, had to be a clear and direct expression of the new medical centre at Blackthorn. This was the broad framework for the brief.

Warmth of the surroundings was required to create a personal, caring experience where social relationships could be encouraged to develop. Loneliness in society hinders the healing process and every effort was made to create a social building that brought to expression the care of one human being for another, a building where the sense of 'self' could emerge.

On entering the Blackthorn Medical Centre one is met by an open waiting area with modulated volumes formed by various ceiling heights, so that the introvert and extrovert can feel comfortable. A reception desk is discreetly positioned, but accessible, with vertical circulation and the two wings with consultation and therapy rooms clearly visible so that the building and its parts do not remain a mystery.

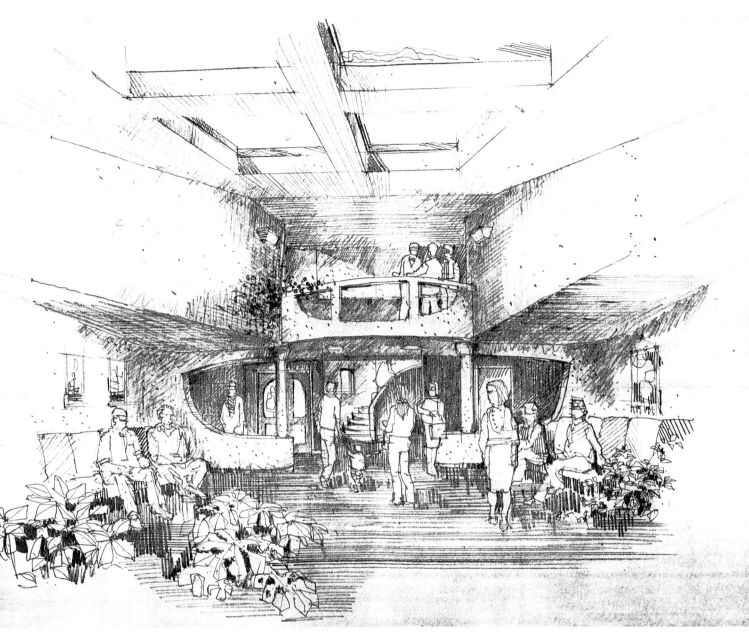

Directly beyond the waiting area is a garden which is embraced by the building. At the centre of the garden is a water cascade. The cascade is composed of a series of sculptured, dish-like forms which bring to expression the nature of water and its archetypal state. Water flows in rhythms, meanders and spirals through cascades. This is another attempt to re-activate man's unconscious relationship to nature.

The waiting area was designed to be large enough also for use for lectures, concerts, exhibitions and activities which arise out of the community experience. The curved bridge on the first floor forms a balcony for additional seating.

It is hoped that the building and its environment will bring inspiration and contribute to the process of healing. As Rudolph Steiner has emphasized:

Man can only experience true harmony of soul when what his soul knows to be its most valuable thoughts, feelings and impulses are mirrored for his senses in the form and colours of his surroundings.

The experience and direction of such centres as the Blackthorn Medical Centre, together with the emerging trends in the United States suggest the creation of appropriate environments for the

△ *Blackthorn Medical Centre Architect's sketch showing concept of open waiting area with modulated volumes formed by various ceiling heights. Architects and illustration: Camphill Architects, Aberdeen, Scotland.*

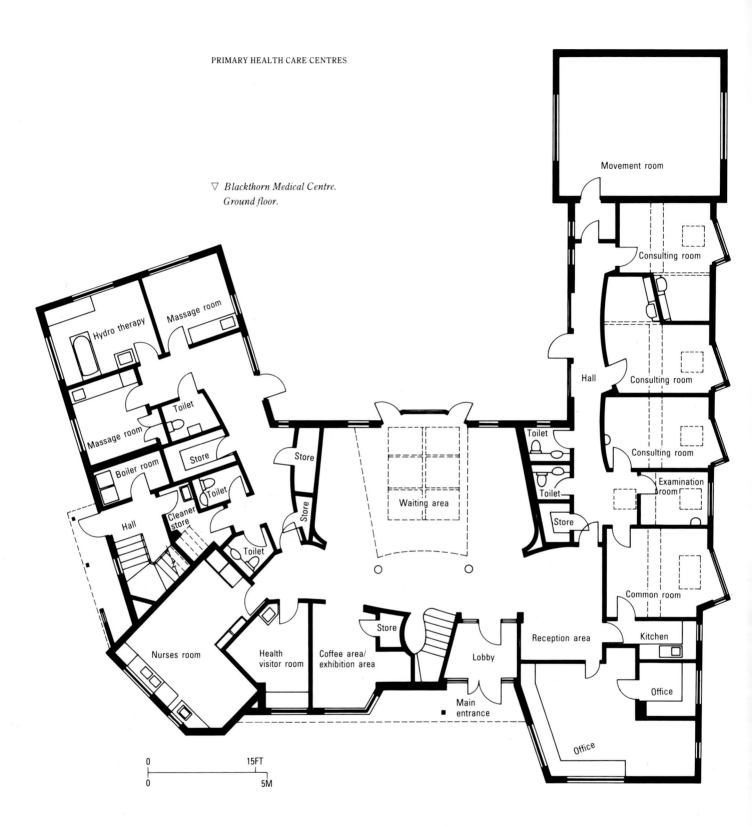

▽ *Blackthorn Medical Centre.*
  Ground floor.

Movement room

Consulting room

Consulting room

Hall

Consulting room

Examination room

Hydro therapy

Massage room

Toilet

Store

Massage room

Store

Waiting area

Toilet

Boiler room

Store

Toilet

Common room

Store

Hall

Toilet

Cleaner store

Reception area

Kitchen

Toilet

Nurses room

Health visitor room

Coffee area/ exhibition area

Store

Lobby

Office

Main entrance

Office

0   15FT

0   5M

health, therapy and well-being of a person as a whole, rather than merely treating patients for medical illness.

As such the future may not be far removed from the ideals of the Peckham and Finsbury health centres, which ran within such a framework over half a century ago.

Perhaps the social/political climate of the 1990s will be more responsive to these ideals within a framework of a greater awareness of health care, the promotion of fitness and the dangers of an over-reliance upon pharmaceutical drugs for certain conditions. After all, both medicine and architecture are tending to place less of an emphasis on high technology, and instead are becoming more sensitive to the needs of the human condition, the environment and earth's finite resources.

▽ *Blackthorn Medical Centre. First floor.*

▽ *Architect's sketch proposal for Blackthorn Medical Centre. The new building's aim is to continue and expand the innovative field of work of its group of medical and health practitioners, reflected within a healing and holistic approach to primary care. Architects: Camphill Architects, Aberdeen, Scotland.*

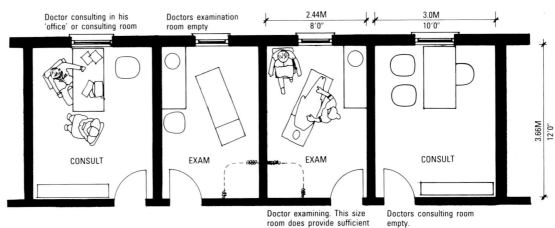

Doctor consulting in his 'office' or consulting room

Doctors examination room empty

2.44M / 8'0" 3.0M / 10'0"

3.66M / 12'0"

CONSULT EXAM EXAM CONSULT

Utilization = 50% of rooms
Clinical rooms provide too nett a fit restricting potential for flexibility over time.

Doctor examining. This size room does provide sufficient space for escort for patient or for doctor to take notes.

Doctors consulting room empty.

▷ Sketch layout indicating possible arrangement for larger but shared room activity of examination, rather than each doctor having his own, yet smaller, examination room.

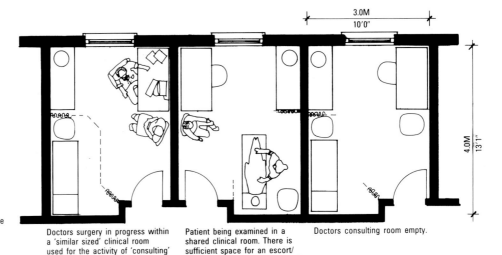

3.0M / 10'0"

4.0M / 13'1"

Utilization = 66% of rooms
Rooms of similar size more flexible for change of use over time

Doctors surgery in progress within a 'similar sized' clinical room used for the activity of 'consulting'

Patient being examined in a shared clinical room. There is sufficient space for an escort/assistant/student. Doctor may also continue to 'consult' or 'interview' in same room.

Doctors consulting room empty.

Architecture and medicine

Health care is a dynamic process. Architecture for health consequently has to strive for shells for lively continuous changing organisms.[11]

There is only one aspect of the future for primary health care that we can safely predict, and that is it will be unpredictable.
Professor Raymond Moss

We are living yesterday's future and tomorrow's history. The only tangible commodity we can therefore deal with is the present. For primary health care buildings standing on the threshold of the future, can we change our conversation from attempting to define the buildings of the future too closely to instead creating environments which will simply allow the future to happen? that is, to avoid designing buildings today that will not restrict the potential of tomorrow.

This final section of the book has been written within the framework of a debate (or forum) held with those who research, design and use primary health care facilities. Those who have contributed to this debate are therefore quoted directly.

184

Buildings are expensive: they take a long time to build and are rarely updated or modified quickly enough to respond to changing needs. In short, buildings often suffer from an incurable time-lag in that they do not reflect where we are but rather tell us where we were when the facility was originally designed.

This factor is critical to primary care facilities, for, like an amoeba, organizational demands of both staff and patients are constantly changing and evolving. Unfortunately, the building shells have tended to be unable to change in unison over time, resulting therefore in a constant mis-match between demand and supply in a nation's primary health care building stock.

Future change is inevitable. However, the danger is that architects and their clients will only consider the negative aspects of planning for the future. A building will flex only so far. Perhaps one way to anticipate future change is to reverse the line of thought, and instead to examine those aspects which we may feel safe in assuming will not change.

Dr Ruth Cammock, who was both an architect and general practitioner, addressed herself to this very matter during her research in the early 1970s, still highly relevant for the 1990s. She described the unchanging aspects of future buildings for primary health care. With this innovative approach to the problem her work has provided us with some important clues as how best to plan our future primary care buildings. It is also an important reminder to architects and their clients that the basics of providing a suitable building shell to accommodate the delivery of primary care must be recognized prior to contemplating future developments. It is worthwhile examining those basics which will not – and perhaps should not – change in the future.

Dr Cammock proposed that so long as building is used for primary care it will house health care staff and their patients. The patients will be the people visiting/living in the facility, and the staff will include both professional and supporting personnel. Although the sizes of these groups and individual

roles within them may change, their relationship to each other and the needs of their members as human beings will probably remain much the same throughout the building's life time.

Progressive change

Any change of use which continues in the same direction will eventually enforce change in the structure of the building. Architects of future primary health care premises should aim to postpone this need for structural change. Although we cannot see far into the future, much can be achieved by keeping options open. Primary health care buildings should, therefore, be planned so that they can expand if necessary without disrupting the original facilities.

Bruce Bonine AIA, of the NBBI Group, writing in the AIA Memo (September 1990)[12] argued that more attention will also be given to planning strategies which create an 'orderly, adaptability pattern' for growth and change. Bonine further explains this by suggesting the zoning of 'soft' low-tech users adjacent to fast growing high-tech users, thereby allowing future expansion at a relatively low cost. Also suggested is creation of 'surge' zones which allow a building's perimeter or even as landscaped courtyard zones within the core of the facility's footprint to allow future expansion for fast growing departments or the unpredictable growth of departments affected by new modes of care or new medical technologies.

You have to ask yourself whether you need to move walls at all. Most of the spaces within the primary care facility are in the order of approximately 11 sq m to 17 sq m (120–180 sq ft) and these are the spaces that small groups of approximately 2–4 people can fit in to discuss something. this does not necessarily imply moving partitions. Instead we have to move more towards a robust flexibility within primary health care design.
Stephen Gage

Dr Ruth Cammock continued in her work to explain that developments in medicine will change the amount and the kind of equipment used; since some items may decrease while others increase, the building should be planned to remain serviceable throughout considerable changes of this kind.

Bruce Bonine, in his article for the *AIA Memo* (September 1990), also mentions the intentional inclusion of what he calls 'swing space', that is to allow temporary relocation of departments beyond the direct programmatic needs during upgrading/ improvements.

Space as a resource – value for money

When viewed within financial terms, space may indeed be identified as an expensive resource. The effective management of space will therefore need to become an increasingly important factor as information technology cuts loose from the computer rooms and invades the clinical room, as energy costs continue to rise and the politics of the health care environment becomes increasingly complex.
Derek Salter, Care Design Group

Getting value for money out of primary health care space has, of course, always been a puzzle and a concern to operators and architects alike contemplating building new or improved existing practice premises. The continuing energy crunch and the rising costs of building will make the puzzle even more difficult to solve.

We have been contacted by a local bereavement counselling service who also use our group space in our centre. We are also going to allow them to use our consulting suites at times when we are not using them, in order to maximize the resources we have. It's quite clear that whilst it is very nice to have your own consulting room it is not used intensively enough in view of the capital expenditure, so one wants to look to ways of using these rooms for other purposes.
Dr Chris Hindley

Just as a financial company will scrutinize its resources, so in the future medical staff administrators and architects will need to cast a more critical eye over existing wasted circulation, uneven densities and space use.

How can these principles of 'space planning' be interpreted by health care managers and their

architects for tomorrow's primary care buildings? Certainly no building owner/user will know more about this future to instruct an architect to design a primary health care facility that will last for five, let alone 50 years. Planning horizons are too close: targets come and go like telegraph poles seen from the windows of a fast moving train. The goal will therefore be to devise building programmes that track a middle way that mediates between instantaneous needs and long-term flexibility.

John Weeks, an architect with considerable experience in the design of hospitals, in a paper on 'Design strategy for flexible health sciences'[13] describes the concept of the indeterminate building. The structure or planning of such a building, he argues, would not dominate or restrict any present pattern of work. Professor Raymond Moss, of MPA, has explained how Weeks' prescription was not to design as if he final building was the end of the matter, but to allow the building to contain possibilities of continuous adjustment to reality during the lifetime of its occupation.

One should try and produce sets of rooms that allow themselves to be furnished and used in a variety of ways. If such rooms can be as non-specific in that respect as possible it can then lead to a variety of modes of use. Flexibility is the key aspect.
John Allan

Following Weeks' own work, Dr Cammock looked into the utilization of consulting suites and treatment rooms to assess the effective utilization of the various spaces within a health centre.[14]

In the health centres studied a major part of each building was taken up by rooms which were used for consultations, interviews, examination and/or treatment. These rooms were labelled by the design guidance which formed the programme/ brief for the building as either:

- Consulting rooms
- Examination rooms
- Interview rooms
- Treatment rooms
- Dental surgery and recovery room
- Chiropody room

186

Most of the published guidance recommended a different sort of space for each of these labelled areas. However, as a result of the research which involved observing the activities of each of the rooms it became apparent that in essence each activity carried out in these labelled areas demanded a very similar sort of space. For example, a social worker interviewing a patient was really the same activity as the doctor consulting his/hers/ A nurse giving an injection in an examination room was really the same activity as a nurse obtaining a blood specimen in the treatment area. Another point was that each activity demanded a high degree of visual and audio privacy to prevent overhearing and overseeing. It was also found that a similar number of people usually occupied this room, i.e. one member of staff, one escort/assistant/student, and one patient. Many of the centres studied were in fact having problems after a change in staffing or operational policy or when a service had been added or withdrawn, because they were unable successfully to adapt these labelled rooms to other functions. The problem was further aggravated in many of these rooms by fixed equipment and furniture.

At the time that the research was undertaken, official design guidance recommended the spaces for the following rooms (DHSS Design Guide (Revised) 1974):

Room	Area (m²)	Area (ft²)
Consulting room	11.00	118.00
Family doctor's consulting room	13.00	140.00
Speech therapy	14.00	151.00
Nursing staff interview	11.00	118.00
Chiropody	11.00	118.00
Dental surgery (principal local health authority)	14.50	156.00
Recovery (local health authority)	9.50	102.00
Dental surgery and office (local health authority)	16.50	178.00
Dental surgery (GP)	12.50	135.00
Dental surgery (subsidiary GP)	9.50	102.00
Treatment	17.00	183.00
Examination room	5.00	54.00
Family doctor's examination room	6.50	70.00

This table shows that the various areas are very similar, yet it appeared irrational that a building which should be designed to permit maximum flexibility in use and future use (as design guidance often advocates) should have the millstone of different areas for each label around its neck, even though the activities that go under these labels are virtually the same. For example, no logical reason could explain why the examination activities of a family doctor involved 1.5 sq m (16 sq ft) more space than a National Health Service doctor, even though both types of doctor teach.

In the *Community Health Centres: Design In Use Study*, commissioned by the North East Thames Regional Health Authority,[15] this aspect was further examined by the author who dealt in particular with the use of consulting and examination rooms.

The examination rooms within the centres studies were one of the most under-used spaces in the building. It seemed rather an elaborate provision that each consulting room should have its own examination room. In practice, most of the doctors held their surgeries at different times. As a result there was always a vacant examination room throughout the day.

When in use, many doctors complained that they were too small. For example, they were unable to gain access to both sides of the examination couch. Conditions became very cramped when a third person (i.e. nurse, student or escort, etc.) was also in the room. Thus from studying the various centres and observing the activities that are concerned with the design of health centres, it was noted that what was really needed was fewer but larger spaces for the activities of patient examination and area similar to that for consulting would be far more efficient.

The advantages associated with this are:
• Greater flexibility in use – as a room which may be used for examination it can also be used for consulting/interviewing, etc.
• The building is more economically used, with doctors sharing examination rooms. Every two consulting rooms has one room which may be used for examination.

• The building becomes cheaper to construct in that it demands less duplication of services, one larger shared room for examination instead of two smaller spaces.

It was not until 1991 that official UK government design guidance finally recognized and recommended this concept.[16] If space as a resource is to become more precious, then even the American model of the doctors' accommodation comprising an office plus a multiple examination room may need to be re-thought.

Future design concepts for primary health care facilities will perhaps move away from the traditional concept of a building with a particular set of functions towards the idea of a building as an envelope, integrating particular functions more loosely.

The architect's task will therefore be merely to provide a framework, a sort of kit of parts, in which people will be able to do what they want.

There is a case for looking at plans which are capable of having spaces and rooms which are valuable for a variety of different uses over time.
John Allan

We must therefore plan to achieve a loose, rather than a net fit.
Professor Raymond Moss

Primary health care buildings planned too precisely for today's needs will stand little chance of adapting to the needs of tomorrow. However, facilities which contain rooms of approximately the same size, which roughly fit today's users, will stand a far better chance of roughly fitting tomorrow's users and will certainly represent better value for money over time. This is perhaps the key to providing indeterminate primary health care premises.

Re-use of existing building stock
Planning concepts will also have to take account of the buildability of future projects and the constraints of our existing building stock and future sites for new buildings.

Although previous design guidance and commercial considerations favoured new buildings, it is impractical and, on a global scale, no longer cost nor energy efficient automatically to think in terms of new buildings for primary care premises. Existing building stock can be recycled to provide cost-effective accommodation for primary health care. The architectural profession has traditionally put a huge premium and devoted most of its prestige to the design of new buildings. Of course this is, and no doubt will remain, important. Other kinds of design activity and the question of how existing buildings can be designed for better use have sadly been neglected, and both will need to be rectified in the future.

There is an enormous amount of design (useful and socially relevant) that is possible without actually having to build a new building at all. A new building should be no more than a device tactic, something you would have to do only on occasions. The design of new buildings for primary health care, particularly within inner city (Fourth World) environments, should therefore form only part of the overall building programme. Techniques for reusing existing building stock will therefore need to be further researched and developed.

Problems rarely occur overnight. By the time a project team is assembled they are dealing with a problem – particularly in existing facilities – that may have been apparent for several months of even years. This therefore focuses on the need for a project team to maintain an on-going relationship with a health facility; regular evaluation programmes to test and define how well a facility is working against the criteria from which it was originally designed. The goal to which designers and managers of health facilities in primary care should be working towards is not just that of solving problems but, more importantly, anticipation of problems, so that solutions can be planned for and built into long-term budgets. We are all very familiar with the very sound advice that preventive medicine and promotion of wellness can avoid the onset of serious illness and save both ourselves and the nation huge expense on acute care. Perhaps we can therefore seriously begin to think about preventive architecture so as to develop a health facility with a planned and co-ordinated programme of development over time, to try and anticipate change rather than just respond or react to it. Long-range planning does not necessarily imply that every solution is resolved by a building. It could mean a revised management structure or replacement or upgrading of equipment and materials. The architect is therefore moving away from merely being the provider of new or upgraded buildings, towards one who understands how best those buildings can be used, being sensitive to staff and patient needs over time: from space planner to space manager.

Energy consciousness raising

Energy is expensive and is most likely to continue to be so. It is also, in absolute terms, becoming a scarce commodity. These two factors will have increasing financial implications for the users of future primary health care buildings. Lighting is an extremely significant user of energy because of its prime use of electricity. Heating is another large user, though alternative fuels are available.

Energy-conscious design must become an increasingly exact science in primary health care buildings, as it has already become in office design.

The pursuance of any energy-efficient primary care buildings relies, to a great extent, upon health administrators' and users' ability to use, control and manage energy at the point of use in particular when different sets of users work in the facility at different times. Whilst the design team can create building envelopes that will effectively retain heat, energy consumption rests largely with users having the ability to monitor and control its use. The concepts of defensible space, where users can identify the spaces they can control, can be applied to energy. That is, defensible energy, enabling users autonomy and responsibility in relating energy use to localized rather than centralized control.

Therefore as with the utilization of space, energy use involves capital expenditure and has consequences on revenue. The project team will need to determine the most efficient and effective means of providing lighting, heating and cooling within the budget. Decisions will also need to be made as to the specification of the building shell in terms of insulation standards. Savings made in capital costs may well produce further expense in the long term. Because of the variety of users within a primary health care facility it will be necessary to monitor and evaluate how energy is being used almost within the framework of a financial audit.

New technology

Despite all predictions made since the late 1960s concerning the use of computers in primary health care, the impact of new office technology has still been underestimated.

When we first started thinking about our new practice premises we did allow space for a computer, but did not envisage the extent to which the use of computers would influence our way of working or the spaces we would need to accommodate its use. Because this building was designed to adapt to such unforeseen circumstances, we have managed to introduce computers and make minor modifications to the building without too much disruption or construction cost.
Dr Chris Hindley

During the last five years computer technology has evolved faster than ever before, and apparently far faster than anything design imagination can cope with.

The temptation for the future, seductive as ever (especially to both architects and medical staff), will be to go along with the prevalent myth that computer gadgets will solve all ills and to abandon thinking for fashion. Fashion will not be good enough. Images are important to architects, but images need to be continuously and rigorously checked. The full impact of the computer technology revolution is still yet to be felt. In the future we will need to harness its strength and avoid its pitfalls.

A major problem encountered with information technology systems is their incompatibility across different products. As the industry becomes more sophisticated, so greater compatibility will allow for a more simplified means of upgrading or assembling different packages of systems.

At one level it must be accepted that the advance in information technology will continue to accelerate. The key will be to integrate a computer system with the possibility of upgrading and expanding, in preference to a programme of constant replacement.

Towards a conclusion: briefing is the core

Despite an unpredictable future, certain clearly definable issues have emerged which architects and their clients will need to address, so that the projects on the drawing board respond to the demands of primary health care into the next century. A fundamental issue is the process by which the next generation of these building is designed. Primary health care is witnessing tremendous change on an international scale.

Architects will need to compile more rigorous yet flexible briefs/programmes in order to take account of present and anticipated activities. The medical client simply giving the architect a list of rooms required, and their sizes, simply will not do.
Joe Jordan

The onus will be on the architect to ask questions and compile data, and on the client bodies to encourage a greater emphasis on the brief for the project.

It is important to get close in a real sense to one of the most important primary end users: the doctors and their medical and administrative staff.
Stephen Gage

Briefing (i.e. the preparation of the project programme) is not primarily concerned with sites or buildings. It is ideally concerned with understanding organizations, activities and how

that organization functions and can change. Essentially it is a two-way learning process, where the architect and client body learn to understand and utilize each other's particular skills and experience to produce a satisfactory design solution. It is therefore important that the prime users – the medical and administrative staff – are considered 'members' of the design team. Briefing should not be seen as a rigid set of instructions, but rather a statement of intent which should develop with the design.

It cannot be assumed that design guidance will automatically lead to better designed buildings. Past examples of health centres in the United Kingdom, and design according to design guidance data, bear witness to this. Design guidance is often out of date by the time it is published. It is usually a document of the past, and not the future.
Stephen Gage

As a two-way learning process, the architect needs to learn not only about how the medical and administrative staff will work but also needs to take the initiative to enlighten the doctors about the design possibilities and to expand their terms of reference. Often the briefing process will be a period of structuring a client-body's own thoughts and aspirations within a framework that can be communicated to the architect and then interpreted within that design framework.

It is important to note that the preparation of a design activity programme (the brief) is an on-going process, and that as the design evolves from the conceptual to the specific it should be generated through an on-going dialogue between architects and the primary care team users.
Derek Salter, Care Design Group.

Design work, however detailed, should be continually tested to ensure that it will suitably fit the practice organizations and requirements.

Depending on how and where medical staff have been practising, their own mode of working may change greatly when they move to their new building. We have worked with a group of doctors who previously were working from sub-standard accommodation, the most charitable

description of which would be that is was 'cosy' in that you almost had to climb over someone or something to get anywhere. They did not really know how their operation was going to change. However, through briefing and open discussions possibilities became apparent that would not have been fully realized had the design been frozen at too early a stage.
John Allan

Briefing is therefore important because it will be the only way the architect can begin to comprehend the complexities of primary health care and to understand how future change will affect the design proposal. It will also provide a precious opportunity for the client group to co-ordinate their thoughts and plan ahead; to assemble their requirements within a structured format as far as how they would wish to work together in terms of operational policies, management and patient care services.

Whatever the system or procurement that different types of primary health care buildings involve, and whatever financing arrangements there are, there isn't really any substitute or short cut to avoid formulating in detail a brief with the people who are preferably going to use the building.
Justin De Syllas

Initially the briefing process should not be seen as a rigid set of instructions, but rather as a statement of intent which should develop with the design process. Generally a brief should include the following five stages of development:

1 The present situation, organization and practice premises.
It is important at this early stage for the architect to become familiar and sensitive to the practice organization, i.e. premises, personnel and how they function. This will sensitize the architect to the current premises' problems and needs.
2 Checklist of basic information.
Here, the architect will establish and become familiar with the type of work and services the practice intends to offer, together with the number of projected staff and patients who will use the building. Often the practice is given the chance to think beyond merely the number of rooms it

requires, imagining instead how – in an ideal world – they would wish to practise and what type of building facilities they would ideally seek. Whilst of course the real world of financial constraints of the cost rent scheme plus the limitations of any site will inevitably restrict what at the end of the day is actually possible, it is still worthwhile taking some imaginative leaps during these early stages. Dr Lorraine Hiatt, a consultant on environmental design and ageing, has called this process 'dreaming with your feet on the ground'.[17] That is, to take ideas on board and, if necessary, reject them as a 'flushing out' of ideas between the practice partners and their staff.
3 Testing the information.
From the information obtained, the architect can prepare some initial sketch plan proposals. These often serve as a framework upon which to discuss more detailed aspects of the design. A sketch design, however preliminary, can often act as a catalyst and bring to light information which doctors may have difficulty in describing in abstract terms. The sketch design will also focus more clearly on the project's possibilities and restrictions in terms of financial constraints and the restrictions of a particular site. The agreed sketch plan proposals could also involve:

- Consultation with the health authorities to gain their opinion as to the suitability of the site building in relation to the terms and conditions of health codes, etc.
- The seeking of outline planning permission (zoning) or detailed planning permission if specifically required by the local planning authority (in the case of existing buildings).
- Estimate of costs.
- An outline specification.

4 Learning from each other.
From these initial plans more detailed proposals will be prepared. As a two-way process the architect will need not only to learn about how the doctors and their staff work, but will also need to take the initiative to involve the doctors in the design to ensure that they are aware of all major decisions.

5 Developing the design.

It is important to note that briefing is an on-going process, and that as the design evolves from the conceptual site plans to the specific details drawings there should be a continuous dialogue between the architect and the practice to ensure that, as far as possible, the original aims and intentions of the practice are being successfully translated into the proposed design solution.

Briefing is, therefore, about communication. The most successful primary health care centre projects have often been the results of a collaborative approach between the architect and the practice.

Surviving future change

For both financial and social reasons resources will continue to be directed away from centralized institutional care towards more locally and community-based centres. The importance of an adequate primary health care infrastructure will therefore become even more relevant to the goal of health for all. The time is therefore now ripe for the injection of new ideas and a more structured approach for the development of a primary health care facility planning. However only by sharing our experiences to exchange ideas and information, can we build together a richer fund of knowledge and expertise with which to meet the challenge of the future. We must explore opportunities for greater co-operation across the professions and across the diverse bureaucracies especially a partnership between primary and secondary care to enrich the palette from which new ideas and innovations can be created.

Finally, architecture for primary health care in terms of the services and activities that it accommodates cannot be discussed in isolation. It is merely part of a wider debate to achieving the objectives of the World Health Organisation's Alma-Ata Declaration, that is, to improve the health of all nations so that by the year 2000 reasonable health conditions will prevail throughout the world.

Martin S. Valins

Key points and checklist to allow future change:

1 It is important that at an early stage the architect becomes sensitive to the practice/facility/organization (in terms of its existing premises, personnel and how the facility functions).

2 Establish a checklist of basic information to achieve a familiarity with the type of work and services the facility intends to offer in the future. This will include anticipated numbers of staff, patients, plus information systems, range of services and activities.

3 Use initial sketch plan diagrams to test, evaluate and update both basic information and design drawings.

4 During initial planning stages (however conceptual) consult at the earliest possible opportunity with relevant health authorities, zoning/planning authorities and fire regulative personnel to ensure that their advice and opinion are taken on board and can therefore be incorporated at an early stage to ensure compliance.

5 Utilize sketch plan proposals as a vehicle for information exchange between architect and project team plus, where appropriate, other intended users for new or improved facilities.

6 Maintain the process of information exchange and testing throughout the design process. Test the designs against the unexpected. Take imaginative leaps into the future, keeping feet firmly on the ground, and test whether the design survives the journey. If the design can 'fly' with you – albeit in concept – then it may stand a good chance of surviving future change.

7 Avoid the pitfalls of designing too closely to an exact fit simply to satisfy the idiosyncrasies of a staff member or a department. Despite whatever constraints there may be, try to inspire the project team to adopt the principle of long life, loose fit, low cost.

8 Wherever possible, attempt to make as many of the clinical spaces which will be used for similar activities to a common size. This will allow for flexibility, change and interchange of personnel staff areas without the need for structural alterations.

192

9 Allow 'surge zones' around the perimeter of the building, or as courtyards, for unpredictable future expansion. Try to zone soft low-tech users adjacent to fast-growing high-tech users so that the facility remains serviceable throughout an expansion programme, if required.

10 From day one, consider options for energy use; building budgets will need to take account of both capital and revenue expenditure in terms of the specification of the building shell and the sophistication of the energy system used and its management control system.

11 Once the project team is assembled for the proposed facility, attempt to maintain an on-going relationship with that team even after the facility has been completed. Undertake regular and on-going evaluations of how the spaces are being utilized and how the building is functioning so as to anticipate future change rather than responding or reacting to it.

References

1. Wright, G. (1987) Senior living facilities provide range of options. *Building & Design Construction* February 50.

2. Lubbock, J. (1985 A patient revolution. *The Architect's Journal*, 16th October 63–103.

3. CM 249 (1987) Promoting Better Health. *The Government's Programme for Improving Primary Health Care*, HMSO, London.

4. *Report of the enquiry into London's Health Service, Medical Education and Research*, (1992) HMSO, London.

5. SPRI (1984) *Primary Care in Progress*, SPRI, Stockholm.

6. Jarman, B. (1981) A survey of primary care in London, Royal College of General Practitioners, London.

7. Acheson, D. (1981) *Primary Health Care in Inner London* London.

8. Bosanquet, N., Laing, W. and Propper, C. (1990) *Elderly Consumers in Britain: Europe's Poor Relations?* Laing & Buisson Publications Ltd., London.

9. Ibid.

10. McKahan, D. (1990) *Vision 2000: Health Care Design*, American Institute of Architects (Memo September 1990), Washington D.C., USA.

11. Reference and background paper of the IUA-PHG to World Health Organization-DSHS P.21/522/5 – regarding experience and findings of architecture for health in view of the WHO's strategy Health for All by the Year 2000. IUA Public Health Group, BDA, Bonn, Germany, 26th April 1989, 6.

12. Bonine, B. (1990) *Vision 2000: Health Care Design*, American Institute of Architects, (Memo September 1990), Washington D.C. USA.

13. Weeks, J. and Best, C. (1970) *Design Strategy for Flexible Health Sciences Facilities*, Institute on Hospital Design, American Hospitals Association, Chicago, USA.

14. Cammock, R. (1977) *Utilization of Consulting Suites in Health Centres*, Medical Architecture Research Unit, London.

15. Valins, M.S. (1975) *Community Health Centres: Design in Use Study*, North East Thames Regional Health Authority, London.

16. Health Building Note 46. (1991) 'General medical practice premises for the provision of primary care services': NHS Estates. HMSO, London.

17. Hiatt, L. (1989) Taken from lecture at the American Association of Homes for the Ageing's annual conference, Baltimore, Maryland, USA, October.

Bibliography

There have been numerous distinguished papers and publications on the subject of design for health care. Below is a selection of the publications which I found most useful and relevant while researching *Primary Health Care Centres*

Alford, T.W. (1979) *Facility Planning, Design and Construction of Rural Health Centres*, Ballinger Publishing Company, Cambridge, Mass, USA.

Beales, J.G. (1978) *Sick Health Centres*, Pitman Medical, London.

Bosker, G. (1987) Architecture as an asset in health care, *architecture*, January, 48–53.

Bryant, J.H. *et al.* (1976) *Community Hospitals and Primary Care*, Ballinger Publishing Company, Cambridge, Mass, USA.

Cammock, R. (1981) *Primary Health Care Buildings*, The Architectural Press, London.

Conference of Missionary Societies (1975) *A Model Health Centre*, working party report by 1972 Medical Committee, Conference of Missionary Societies in Great Britain and Ireland, London.

Cox, A. and Groves, P. (1990) *Hospitals and Health Care Facilities*, Butterworth Architecture, London.

Davies, C. (1988) Architecture of Caring. *the Architectural Review*, **1096**, 15–17.

Dudley Hunt, W. (1960) Hospital, clinics & health centers, in *Architectural Record*, F.W. Dodge Corporation. USA.

Gaskie, M. (1985) Re-inventing the hospital, *Architectural Record*, October 1985, USA, 127–132.

Goldsmith, S. (1984) *Designing for the Disabled*, RIBA Publications, London.

Hannay, P. and Hallett, K. (1987) Doctors on the street and preventative medicine. *the Architects Journal*, **186**(38), 127–132.

Havlicek, P.L. (1985) *Medical Groups in the USA 1984*, American Medical Association, Chicago, USA.

Hoglund, J.D. (1985) *Housing the Elderly*, Van Nostrand Reinhold, New York, USA.

International Union of Architects Public Health Group (1989) Reference and background paper of the UIA-PHG to WHO-DSHS District Health Systems, 26th April 1989.

Knight III, C. (1987) Designing for the health care process and market place, *Architecture*, **76**(1), 48–52.

Malkin, J. 91982) *The design of Medical & Dental Facilities*, Van Nostrand Reinhold, New York, USA.

Malkin, J. (1990) *Medical and Dental Space Planning for the 1990s*, Van Nostrand Reinhold, New York, USA.

Marks, L. (1987) *Primary Health Care on the Agenda: A Discussion Document*, The King's Fund Institute, London.

Marks, L. (1988) *Promoting Better Health?: An Analysis of the Government's Programme for Improving Primary Health Care*, The King's Fund Institute, London.

Paine, L.H.W. and Siem Tjam, F. (1988) *Hospitals and the Health Care Revolution*, World Health Organization, Geneva, Switzerland.

Pearce, I.H. and Crocker, L.H. (1985) *The Peckham Experiment: A Study of The Living Structure of Society*, Scottish Academic Press, Edinburgh.

Pritchard, P. (1981) *Manual of Primary Health Care*, 2nd edn, Oxford University Press, London.

Redstone, L.G. (ed.) (1978) Hospital and Health Care Facilities, in *Architectural Record*, McGraw-Hill Book Company, USA.

Reizenstein Carpman, J. *et al.* (1986) *Design that Cares*, American Hospital Publishing Inc., Washington DC, USA.

Robinson, R. (1990) *Competition and Health Care: A Comparative Analysis of UK Plans and US Experience*, The King's Fund Institute, London.

Rostenberg, B. (1987) *Design Planning for Free-standing Ambulatory Care Facilities*, American Hospital Association, Chicago, USA.

Sahl, R.J. (1986) Das Krankenhaus: Wanglungen in Anlange und Betrieb. *Deusches Krnakenhausinstitut*, Germany, No. 94, March. (German Hospital Institute in Co-operation with the University of Dusseldorf).

Seliger, M. (1986) *Health for all in Finland*, Laakintohallitus ja Teki jat, Tampere.

The Swedish Planning and Rationalization Institute of the Health and Social Services (SPRI) (1984) *Primary Health Care in Progress*. SPRI, Stockholm, Sweden.

Stallibrass, A. (1989) *Being Me And Also Us: Lessons from the Peckham Experiment*, Scottish Academic Press, Edinburgh.

Stone, P. (1980) *British Hospital and Health Care Buildings*, Architectural Press, London.

Valins, M. (1975) *Community Health Centres*, North East Thames Regional Health Authority, London.

Valins, M. (1990) *Surgery Design Update 1990*, MV&A Research, London.

World Health Organization (1985) *Targets for Health for All: Targets in Support for the European Strategy for Health for All*, World Health Organization Regional Office for Europe, Copenhagen, Denmark.

Wider reading

Although not architectural the following is recommended to those approaching the design of health care buildings which relate to the specific needs of certain conditions and disorders.

Hunger Strike: the Anorexic's Struggle as a Metaphor for our Age by Susie Orbach, 1986, Faber & Faber, London and Boston. Essential reading giving sympathetic and sensitive insight to anorexia nervosa/bulimia.

Theory & Treatment of Anorexia Nervosa & Bulimia: Biomedical, Sociocultural & Psychological Perspectives, ed. Steven W. Emmett, 1985, Brunner-Mazel, New York, USA.

Water & Sexuality by Dr Michel Odent, 1990, Arkana/Penguin, London. Explores the universal attraction that water has for human beings and its use in promoting good health. Useful reading for architects designing maternity/birthing units to understand the importance of providing a pool in which mothers can labour and give birth and the fact that the environment and surroundings have profound effects on the processes of birth and bonding.

The 36-Hour Day by Nancy Mace and Peter Rabins, 1981, Johns Hopkins University Press, USA; 1985, Hodder & Stoughton, UK. Offers insights on Alzheimer's Disease.

Caring for the Person with Dementia published by the Alzheimer's Disease Society, 1158-160 Balham High Road, London SW12 9BN, 1984.

Living with MS by The King's Fund Centre, 1989, London, UK. Helps to understand the emotional difficulties that surround this disorder.

A Personal Exploration by Alexander Burnfield, 1985, Souvenir Pres, UK. A personal account of multiple sclerosis written by a doctor.

Living with AIDS, 1987, Frontliners (55 Farringdon Road, London EXIM 3JB. An invaluable book written by and for people with AIDS.

Living with AIDS & HIV by David Miller, 1987, Macmillan, London. An excellent general account of the virus and its medical and social implications for every reader.

Index

WITHDRAWN

NOT TO BE
TAKEN AWAY

THE LIBRARY
GUILDFORD COLLEGE
of Further and Higher Education

Author Valins Martin

Title Primary Health
Care Centres

Class 725.5 VAL

Accession 71031